Dr Dawn's Guide to Healthy Eating for IBS

Dr Dawn Harper is a GP based in Gloucestershire, working at an NHS surgery in Stroud. She has been working as a media doctor for nearly ten years. Dawn is best known as one of the presenters on Channel 4's award-winning programme *Embarrassing Bodies*, which has run for seven series and two years ago celebrated its hundredth episode. Spin-offs have included *Embarrassing Fat Bodies*, *Embarrassing Teen Bodies* and *Embarrassing Bodies: Live from the clinic*.

Dawn is the presenter of Channel 4's series *Born Naughty?*, one of the doctors on ITV1's *This Morning* and the resident GP on the health hour on LBC radio. She writes for a variety of publications, including *Healthspan*, *Healthy Food Guide* and *NetDoctor*. Her first book, *Dr Dawn's Health Check*, was published by Mitchell Beazley. *Dr Dawn's Guide to Healthy Eating for IBS* is one of five Dr Dawn Guides published by Sheldon Press in 2016. Dawn qualified at London University in 1987. When not working, she is a keen cyclist and an enthusiastic supporter of children's charities. Her website is at <www.drdawn.com>. Follow her on Twitter @drdawnharper.

Azmina Govindji is an award-winning dietitian, international speaker and bestselling author. She is a media spokesperson for the British Dietetic Association, resident dietitian to <www.patient.co.uk>, and a regular contributor to the NHS Choices website. Her television appearances include Sky and ITV breakfast news, *This Morning* as nutritionist (2006–7), *The One Show*, *The Wright Stuff* and BBC's *Watchdog*. She is co-founder of the award-winning RDUK Twitter chats that reach an average of two million people and involve between 60 and 85 expert nutrition participants.

Azmina has written over a dozen books on weight management and diabetes, including cookbooks that are available worldwide. She was chief dietitian to Diabetes UK for eight years and now runs her own nutrition consultancy. She offers authoritative opinion on a range of diet-related topics, and her lively personality and down-to-earth approach help her to simplify scientific dietary principles into realistic hints and tips. Azmina is a mum of two who believes that healthy food can be tasty, and she's passionate about helping people make sense of the hype around diet. Her website is at <www.azminanutrition.com>. Follow her on Twitter @AzminaNutrition or find her on Facebook at Azmina Nutrition.

Overcoming Common Problems Series

Selected titles

A full list of titles is available from Sheldon Press,
36 Causton Street, London SW1P 4ST and on our website at
www.sheldonpress.co.uk

Beating Insomnia: Without really trying
Dr Tim Cantopher

Birth Over 35
Sheila Kitzinger

Breast Cancer: Your treatment choices
Dr Terry Priestman

Chronic Fatigue Syndrome: What you need to know about CFS/ME
Dr Megan A. Arroll

The Chronic Pain Diet Book
Neville Shone

Cider Vinegar
Margaret Hills

Coeliac Disease: What you need to know
Alex Gazzola

Coping Successfully with Chronic Illness: Your healing plan
Neville Shone

Coping Successfully with Hiatus Hernia
Dr Tom Smith

Coping Successfully with Pain
Neville Shone

Coping Successfully with Panic Attacks
Shirley Trickett

Coping Successfully with Prostate Cancer
Dr Tom Smith

Coping Successfully with Shyness
Margaret Oakes, Professor Robert Bor and Dr Carina Eriksen

Coping Successfully with Ulcerative Colitis
Peter Cartwright

Coping Successfully with Varicose Veins
Christine Craggs-Hinton

Coping Successfully with Your Irritable Bowel
Rosemary Nicol

Coping with a Mental Health Crisis: Seven steps to healing
Catherine G. Lucas

Coping with Anaemia
Dr Tom Smith

Coping with Asthma in Adults
Mark Greener

Coping with Blushing
Professor Robert J. Edelmann

Coping with Bronchitis and Emphysema
Dr Tom Smith

Coping with Chemotherapy
Dr Terry Priestman

Coping with Coeliac Disease: Strategies to change your diet and life
Karen Brody

Coping with Difficult Families
Dr Jane McGregor and Tim McGregor

Coping with Diverticulitis
Peter Cartwright

Coping with Dyspraxia
Jill Eckersley

Coping with Early-onset Dementia
Jill Eckersley

Coping with Endometriosis
Jill Eckersley and Dr Zara Aziz

Coping with Envy: Feeling at a disadvantage with friends and family
Dr Windy Dryden

Coping with Epilepsy
Dr Pamela Crawford and Fiona Marshall

Coping with Gout
Christine Craggs-Hinton

Coping with Guilt
Dr Windy Dryden

Coping with Headaches and Migraine
Alison Frith

Coping with Heartburn and Reflux
Dr Tom Smith

Coping with Life after Stroke
Dr Mareeni Raymond

Coping with Liver Disease
Mark Greener

Coping with Memory Problems
Dr Sallie Baxendale

Coping with Obsessive Compulsive Disorder
Professor Kevin Gournay, Rachel Piper and Professor Paul Rogers

Coping with Pet Loss
Robin Grey

Coping with Phobias and Panic
Professor Kevin Gournay

Overcoming Common Problems Series

Coping with Schizophrenia
Professor Kevin Gournay and Debbie Robson

Coping with Stomach Ulcers
Dr Tom Smith

Coping with the Psychological Effects of Cancer
Professor Robert Bor, Dr Carina Eriksen and Ceilidh Stapelkamp

Coping with the Psychological Effects of Illness
Dr Fran Smith, Dr Carina Eriksen and Professor Robert Bor

Coping with Thyroid Disease
Mark Greener

Depression: Why it happens and how to overcome it
Dr Paul Hauck

Depression and Anxiety the Drug-Free Way
Mark Greener

Depressive Illness: The curse of the strong
Dr Tim Cantopher

The Diabetes Healing Diet
Mark Greener and Christine Craggs-Hinton

Dr Dawn's Guide to Brain Health
Dr Dawn Harper

Dr Dawn's Guide to Digestive Health
Dr Dawn Harper

Dr Dawn's Guide to Healthy Eating for Diabetes
Dr Dawn Harper

Dr Dawn's Guide to Healthy Eating for IBS
Dr Dawn Harper

Dr Dawn's Guide to Heart Health
Dr Dawn Harper

Dr Dawn's Guide to Sexual Health
Dr Dawn Harper

Dr Dawn's Guide to Weight and Diabetes
Dr Dawn Harper

Dr Dawn's Guide to Women's Health
Dr Dawn Harper

The Empathy Trap: Understanding antisocial personalities
Dr Jane McGregor and Tim McGregor

Epilepsy: Complementary and alternative treatments
Dr Sallie Baxendale

Fibromyalgia: Your treatment guide
Christine Craggs-Hinton

The Fibromyalgia Healing Diet
Christine Craggs-Hinton

Hay Fever: How to beat it
Dr Paul Carson

The Heart Attack Survival Guide
Mark Greener

Helping Elderly Relatives
Jill Eckersley

Hold Your Head up High
Dr Paul Hauck

The Holistic Health Handbook
Mark Greener

How to Accept Yourself
Dr Windy Dryden

How to Be Your Own Best Friend
Dr Paul Hauck

How to Beat Worry and Stress
Dr David Delvin

How to Eat Well When You Have Cancer
Jane Freeman

How to Listen So that People Talk
Mary Hartley

How to Live with a Control Freak
Barbara Baker

How to Lower Your Blood Pressure: And keep it down
Christine Craggs-Hinton

How to Start a Conversation and Make Friends
Don Gabor

How to Stop Worrying
Dr Frank Tallis

Invisible Illness: Coping with misunderstood conditions
Dr Megan A. Arroll and Professor Christine P. Dancey

The Irritable Bowel Diet Book
Rosemary Nicol

The Irritable Bowel Stress Book
Rosemary Nicol

Jealousy: Why it happens and how to overcome it
Dr Paul Hauck

Living with Autism
Fiona Marshall

Living with Bipolar Disorder
Dr Neel Burton

Living with Complicated Grief
Professor Craig A. White

Living with Eczema
Jill Eckersley

Living with Fibromyalgia
Christine Craggs-Hinton

Living with Hearing Loss
Dr Don McFerran, Lucy Handscomb and Dr Cherilee Rutherford

Living with IBS
Nuno Ferreira and David T. Gillanders

Living with the Challenges of Dementia: A guide for family and friends
Patrick McCurry

Living with Tinnitus and Hyperacusis
Dr Laurence McKenna, Dr David Baguley and Dr Don McFerran

Overcoming Common Problems Series

Living with Type 1 Diabetes
Dr Tom Smith

Losing a Parent
Fiona Marshall

Making Sense of Trauma: How to tell your story
Dr Nigel C. Hunt and Dr Sue McHale

Menopause: The drug-free way
Dr Julia Bressan

Menopause in Perspective
Philippa Pigache

Motor Neurone Disease: A family affair
Dr David Oliver

The Multiple Sclerosis Diet Book
Tessa Buckley

Overcome Your Fear of Flying
Professor Robert Bor, Dr Carina Eriksen and
Margaret Oakes

**Overcoming Anger: When anger helps and
when it hurts**
Dr Windy Dryden

Overcoming Anorexia
Professor J. Hubert Lacey, Christine Craggs-Hinton
and Kate Robinson

Overcoming Anxiety
Dr Windy Dryden

Overcoming Back Pain
Dr Tom Smith

Overcoming Emotional Abuse
Susan Elliot-Wright

Overcoming Fear with Mindfulness
Deborah Ward

**Overcoming Gambling: A guide for problem
and compulsive gamblers**
Philip Mawer

Overcoming Jealousy
Dr Windy Dryden

Overcoming Loneliness
Alice Muir

Overcoming Low Self-esteem with Mindfulness
Deborah Ward

Overcoming Stress
Professor Robert Bor, Dr Carina Eriksen and Dr
Sara Chaudry

Overcoming Worry and Anxiety
Dr Jerry Kennard

**The Pain Management Handbook:
Your personal guide**
Neville Shone

The Panic Workbook
Dr Carina Eriksen, Professor Robert Bor and
Margaret Oakes

**Physical Intelligence: How to take charge of
your weight**
Dr Tom Smith

**Post-Traumatic Stress Disorder: Recovery after
accident and disaster**
Professor Kevin Gournay

Reducing Your Risk of Dementia
Dr Tom Smith

The Self-esteem Journal
Alison Waines

Stammering: Advice for all ages
Renée Byrne and Louise Wright

Stress-related Illness
Dr Tim Cantopher

The Stroke Survival Guide
Mark Greener

Ten Steps to Positive Living
Dr Windy Dryden

**Therapy for Beginners: How to get the best
out of counselling**
Professor Robert Bor, Sheila Gill and Anne Stokes

Think Your Way to Happiness
Dr Windy Dryden and Jack Gordon

**Transforming Eight Deadly Emotions into
Healthy Ones**
Dr Windy Dryden

**The Traveller's Good Health Guide: A guide
for those living, working and travelling
internationally**
Dr Ted Lankester

Treat Your Own Knees
Jim Johnson

Treating Arthritis: More ways to a drug-free life
Margaret Hills

Treating Arthritis: The drug-free way
Margaret Hills and Christine Horner

Treating Arthritis: The supplements guide
Julia Davies

Treating Arthritis Diet Book
Margaret Hills

Treating Arthritis Exercise Book
Margaret Hills and Janet Horwood

Understanding High Blood Pressure
Dr Shahid Aziz and Dr Zara Aziz

Understanding Obsessions and Compulsions
Dr Frank Tallis

**Understanding Yourself and Others: Practical
ideas from the world of coaching**
Bob Thomson

When Someone You Love Has Dementia
Susan Elliot-Wright

**When Someone You Love Has Depression:
A handbook for family and friends**
Barbara Baker

The Whole Person Recovery Handbook
Emma Drew

Overcoming Common Problems

Dr Dawn's Guide to Healthy Eating for IBS

DR DAWN HARPER

Recipes by
AZMINA GOVINDJI

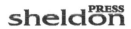

First published in Great Britain in 2016

Sheldon Press
36 Causton Street
London SW1P 4ST
www.sheldonpress.co.uk

Copyright © Dr Dawn Harper 2016
Recipes copyright © Azmina Govindji 2016

All rights reserved. No part of this book may be reproduced or
transmitted in any form or by any means, electronic or mechanical,
including photocopying, recording, or by any information storage and
retrieval system, without permission in writing from the publisher.

The authors and publisher have made every effort to ensure that the
external website and email addresses included in this book are correct and
up to date at the time of going to press. The authors and publisher are not
responsible for the content, quality or continuing accessibility of the sites.

British Library Cataloguing-in-Publication Data
A catalogue record for this book is available from the British Library

ISBN 978–1–84709–390–5
eBook ISBN 978–1–84709–395–0

Typeset by Fakenham Prepress Solutions, Fakenham, Norfolk NR21 8NN
First printed in Great Britain by Ashford Colour Press
Subsequently digitally reprinted in Great Britain

eBook by Fakenham Prepress Solutions, Fakenham, Norfolk NR21 8NN

Produced on paper from sustainable forests

London Borough of Richmond Upon Thames	
RTCA	
90710 000 262 925	
Askews & Holts	
641.563 HAR	£7.99
	9781847093905

Contents

Note to the reader		viii
Introduction		ix
1	Anatomy and physiology of the large bowel	1
2	What is irritable bowel syndrome?	7
3	Food allergy and intolerance	11
4	Diagnosing irritable bowel syndrome	15
5	Managing your irritable bowel syndrome	19
6	FAQs	29
7	The low-FODMAP diet	31
8	**FODMAP-friendly recipes**	**33**
	Be supermarket savvy	34
	Low-FODMAP foods shopping list	35
	Low-FODMAP baking tips	40
	Breakfast ideas	41
	Lunch ideas	43
	Main meals	49
	Vegetarian choices	59
	Time to bake	62
	Hungry between meals?	66
Index		69

Note to the reader

The dietary advice and recipes in this book are intended as a general guide, and not as a substitute for the medical advice of your doctor. Always keep to the advice of your own dietitian and doctor, particularly with respect to any symptoms that may require diagnosis or medical attention.

Introduction

The summer of 1854 was hot. This was before the days of running water in every home, and people were drinking the water they collected from the street taps cold rather than boiling it for tea. There was a dreadful outbreak of diarrhoea in central London during which 89 people died very suddenly. Dr John Snow had the foresight to analyse the link between these deaths. He mapped the locations of the victims' homes and noted that all the families affected were collecting water from a single pump in Broad Street, Soho. In addition, he noted that people nearby, who collected their water from other taps, remained symptom free. A week later Dr Snow persuaded the authorities to remove the handle from the Broad Street pump and the number of infections and deaths fell immediately. He didn't at that stage know why, but he was convinced that the water from that pump was responsible for the outbreak. Today, of course, we know that the multiple deaths were caused by an outbreak of cholera from contaminated water. So why am I telling you this story? Because back in 1854, Dr Snow couldn't prove that the outbreak of diarrhoeal illness was due to infection. He didn't have a microscope to prove the presence of cholera, but he knew it was very real. He was criticized by many at the time for cutting off a valued water supply and lots of people challenged his theory.

There are links here between this story and the emergence of irritable bowel syndrome (IBS) as a diagnosis. Believe it or not, it is not that long ago that there was much debate among specialists as to whether the diagnosis really existed! I remember, when I was at medical school, being told that there were specialists who contested the existence of the condition, believing it to be 'all in the head'. Thankfully, today, just because we can't find abnormalities in blood tests or scans, there is no doubt that IBS exists. It is, in fact, very common and affects as many as one in five British adults and, my guess is, it is even more common that that as many individuals with mild symptoms probably find a way to manage their symptoms without presenting to their GP for diagnosis. It is also a very variable condition. Everyone's story is individual and symptoms can vary hugely from day to day for any one person. IBS is a condition that I encounter every week in surgery and one that can have a significant impact on quality of life. If you are reading this book, you are probably one of those people affected and, so, in this book, I hope to help you to get to know your own disease better so that you can predict flare ups and manage symptoms more effectively. Bottom line? I want you to be in charge of your IBS, and not it in charge of you! I am delighted to have teamed up with Azmina Govindji to provide you with some IBS-friendly recipes that all the family can enjoy.

Dr Dawn's Guide to Healthy Eating for IBS

1

Anatomy and physiology of the large bowel

Irritable bowel syndrome (IBS) is a condition affecting the large bowel and to understand IBS we need to spend some time thinking about what the large bowel does and how it does it. The large bowel (also known as large intestine or colon) is the last part of the intestinal tract and is significantly shorter than the small intestine at approximately 1.5 metres in length. It is called the *large* bowel because it is larger in diameter than the small intestine; about 6–7 cm in diameter for the large bowel and 2.5–3 cm for the small. The large bowel follows on from the small intestine in the bottom right-hand corner of your abdomen at the part of the small bowel called the ileum. As you can see in Figure 1 overleaf, the start of the large bowel is like a sideways 'T' as a small part, called the caecum, hangs down. The appendix comes off the caecum, which is why appendicitis pain is felt low down in the right side of the abdomen. From the ileum, the main part of the large bowel ascends into the top right-hand corner of your abdomen. This, unsurprisingly, is called the ascending colon. Just below the diaphragm, it takes a right-hand bend to run across the top of your abdomen. This is the transverse colon. In the top left-hand corner it takes another right-hand bend to form the descending colon, which goes down to the bottom left-hand corner of your abdomen to become the sigmoid colon and, finally, the rectum.

As with the rest of the gastrointestinal tract, the large bowel wall has four layers and these are:

- *the mucosa*, this is the inner, smooth layer of epithelial tissue that contains the mucus glands that produce mucus to keep the bowel well lubricated and aid the passage of faeces;
- *the submucosa*, this forms a sort of support network for the other layers of bowel wall and contains the blood vessels and nerve fibres supplying the bowel;

1

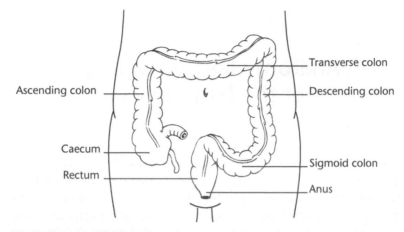

Ascending colon

Transverse colon

Descending colon

Caecum

Rectum

Sigmoid colon

Anus

Figure 1 The large bowel

- *the muscularis*, this is the muscle layer essential for the muscular contractions that propel food and faeces through the gut;
- *the serosa*, this is the outer layer of the bowel and, like the mucosa, it is made of epithelial tissue but the serosa produces a more watery fluid designed to protect the bowel from friction from other organs.

What is the function of the large bowel?

By the time food has reached the large bowel much of the digestive process has taken place in the small bowel and most of the nutrients have already been absorbed, so what arrives in the large bowel is a slurry of mostly digested food known as chyme. The large bowel has three main functions.

- *Digestion* It surprises many people to learn that trillions of good bacteria live in everyone's large bowel – these bacteria weigh around 2 kg in total! These are the gut flora and they help the final process of digestion. The bacteria digest food and fibre that cannot be digested by the small bowel, releasing vital vitamins such as B1, B2, B6, B12 and vitamin K.
- *Absorption* By the time chyme arrives in the large intestine, 80 per cent of the water has been absorbed but the large intestine

can absorb a further 300 ml (about a cup and a half a day) and will also absorb the nutrients provided by the work of the gut flora.

- *Transition* The muscular wall of the large intestine contracts to propel the remaining food, now turning into faeces, along the length of the small gut into the rectum ready for defecation. It takes on average around 47 hours for transit through the large bowel in men and 33 hours in women but, as we all know, transit can at times be much faster and at other times much slower.

What is a normal bowel movement?

I have always said that if I went out on to any high street and asked the first 100 people I bumped into to tell me what a normal period was, I would probably get a pretty accurate answer from the majority (including the men!), but when it comes to bowels we Brits can be rather coy and most of us know very little about anyone's bowel habits other than our own! To a degree that doesn't matter, in that what is important is that we know what is normal for us so that we recognize when things are changing. A normal bowel movement is said to be anything from twice a week to three times a day but perhaps the most important thing is that the stool should be soft, well-formed and easy to pass (see Figure 2 overleaf). You should not have to strain to open your bowels.

How do I know if I am constipated?

It's all about knowing what is normal for you. If you are someone who normally opens your bowels twice a day, then going twice a week could be constipated for you; whereas for someone else that may be their norm. If you are straining to open your bowels, passing very hard motions or feeling that you haven't completely emptied your rectum when you open your bowels then you are probably constipated. Sometimes, if you are very bunged up, you can get some leakage of watery faeces around the blockage, which is easy to mistake as diarrhoea.

Type 1	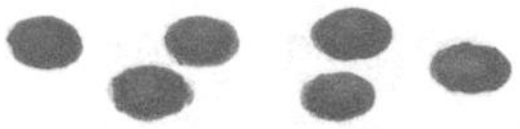	Separate hard lumps, like nuts (hard to pass)
Type 2	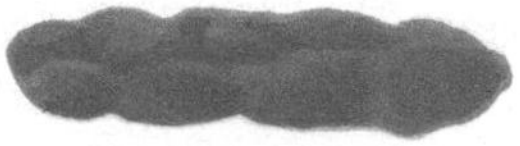	Sausage-shaped but lumpy
Type 3	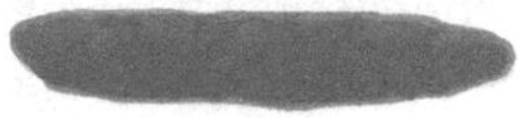	Like a sausage but with cracks on the surface
Type 4	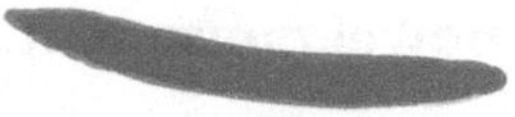	Like a sausage or snake, smooth and soft
Type 5	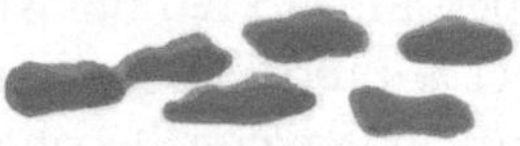	Soft blobs with clear-cut edges
Type 6	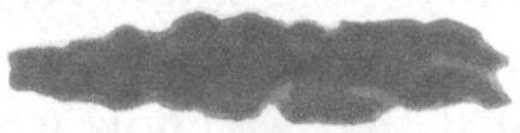	Fluffy pieces with ragged edges, a mushy stool
Type 7	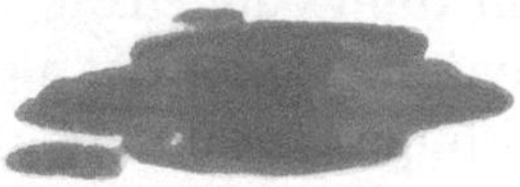	Watery, no solid pieces. Entirely liquid

Figure 2 Bristol stool chart

What are 'red flag' signs?

Doctors talk about 'red flag' signs when they mean symptoms that mustn't be ignored. It is difficult if you have IBS as your bowels will be sensitive and your bowel movements will change but it is important that you get to know your body and recognize symptoms that are not part of your usual IBS. You should see a doctor if:

- you have constipation or diarrhoea persisting for several weeks;
- you have blood in your motions, in the pan or on the paper;
- you lose weight unintentionally;
- you have severe abdominal pain.

What is normal gas production?

It is normal to produce anything between 200 ml and 2 litres of gas a day but as you will no doubt have discovered, some foods may mean you produce significantly more and these include cabbage, onions, pulses and some spices.

Why does my bowel gurgle when I am hungry?

About 12 hours after eating a meal, strong waves of muscular contractions start in the stomach and progress along the full length of the gut. They are sometimes called 'housekeeping movements' and can take as long as 90 minutes to progress along the entire length of the gut. The contractions push air and fluid through the intestine causing what we recognize as gurglings.

Why do I feel sleepy after a large meal?

Eating carbohydrates stimulates the release of a chemical in the brain called serotonin that makes us feel relaxed and contented and is responsible for that postprandial slump!

Why do I get the urge to open my bowels after breakfast?

It is very common for people to feel the need to open their bowels after breakfast and this is because as food enters the digestive tract after a period of relative starvation a wave of contractions moves through the length of the gut. This is called a gastrocolic reflex and, as it pushes faeces towards the rectum and the rectum fills, stretch receptors in the wall of the rectum tell your brain that it needs to empty and you feel the urge to defecate.

2

What is irritable bowel syndrome?

Irritable bowel syndrome (IBS) is a disorder of the function of the bowel. There has been much debate about whether it is due to a heightened awareness of normal contractions of the bowel, or to stronger than normal contractions of the bowel and, to be honest, I suspect there is probably an element of both. Either way, it a very common condition that can affect anyone, although women are twice as likely as men to suffer. It affects as many as one in five of us and can occur at any age, but most people first notice symptoms in their twenties or thirties and often people find that symptoms improve in later life.

What are the symptoms of IBS?

Most people tell me they notice a combination of abdominal pain, bloating and alteration of bowel habits. There are other associated symptoms too, but let's deal with the most common ones first.

- *Pain* The pain of IBS is extremely variable. Some people notice mild abdominal cramps but some women have described the pain as so severe that it reminds them of labour and prevents them from functioning properly. Generally, the pain is cramping in nature and can be felt anywhere in the abdomen. Some people also notice it as back or pelvic pain and in some women IBS can be the cause of pain on sexual intercourse. Typically, IBS patients notice that their symptoms flare up from time to time and then they may go through periods where things improve, but for some the symptoms are relentless and severely affect quality of life.
- *Bloating* Bloating is a common feature of IBS and people often tell me they wake feeling OK, but that during the course of the day they notice increasing distension such that they feel six-months

pregnant and their clothes feel uncomfortably tight. They may also notice more flatulence especially during a flare up.

- *Altered bowel habit* Some people notice a tendency to loose bowel motions and may also experience what we describe as faecal urgency – where they feel the need to open their bowels urgently. Others are more prone to constipation and how we manage your IBS will depend on your individual symptoms so take some time to think about how your IBS affects you before seeing your doctor. It is common to experience a feeling of incomplete emptying after having your bowels open if you have IBS and this is called tenesmus. Some patients may also notice mucus in the motions but there should never be any blood. Rectal bleeding should always be checked out by a doctor to rule out the possibility of rectal cancer. To be fair, the vast majority of cases of bleeding from the back passage are due to benign conditions such as haemorrhoids or small tears in the delicate skin around the anus called fissures, which are not uncommon in IBS patients prone to constipation, but it is better to be safe than sorry.

Some patients also tell me they feel nauseous, or lose their appetite and feel full after eating. Some also develop heartburn or find that they belch more often. There are also non-gut related symptoms including fatigue, headache and muscle pains. Some people report an associated irritable bladder. It is easy to see how persistent and unpleasant symptoms like these can also occasionally also lead to depression.

How do I know that my symptoms are due to IBS and not something more sinister like ovarian cancer?

You may have seen the awareness campaigns urging women not to ignore the possible signs of ovarian cancer and these include persistent:

- bloating
- abdominal or pelvic pain
- feeling full quickly.

A quick scan of the symptoms I have listed above may worry you and, of course, there have been headlines of women presenting with symptoms that have been attributed to IBS and later discovered to be due to ovarian cancer. The crucial word here is *persistent*. Everyone, even those of us who don't suffer with IBS, has felt bloated at some point or has had abdominal pain or felt they simply couldn't eat another thing. IBS sufferers will experience these symptoms frequently but they wax and wane. If you have days when the bloating settles or when you are pain free, this is typical of IBS, but if you are in any doubt see your GP.

3
Food allergy and intolerance

Patients with IBS often ask me if they could be intolerant to a particular food and as you will see below there is a significant overlap in symptoms. I will deal in more depth about excluding food groups and how we assess their impact on symptoms in Chapter 5 but I thought it was important to just highlight the difference between an intolerance and an allergy before we go any further.

Food intolerance (non-allergic or non-immune-mediated food hypersensitivity)

Food intolerances can be difficult to recognize. The symptoms may be vague and the time frames are sometimes not obvious. A food intolerance will not produce antibodies called immunoglobulin E (IgE) to that food like an allergy can. Symptoms often take hours or even days to occur so it can take a long while before the diagnosis is made. Common symptoms include abdominal pain, bloating, diarrhoea or constipation that, as you can see, are very similar to IBS. Patients often describe a feeling of lethargy and poor concentration. Intolerances may occur because of a difficulty digesting a particular food. This can be because of low levels of an enzyme required to break down that food: such as lactase needed to break down lactose, the natural sugar occurring in milk. It is also possible to be intolerant to chemicals in foods such as caffeine, monosodium glutamate and salicylates. Unlike allergies, some people find that they can tolerate small amounts of a particular food but develop symptoms if they overindulge. In fact one theory for why intolerances develop is an overexposure, which may also explain why people with one intolerance go on to develop another because as they change their diet to exclude one food they often end up eating more of another, triggering an intolerance to that. We can't do blood tests for intolerances and I find the best way to identify an intolerance is to keep a detailed food and symptom diary to see if there is a link between diet and symptoms. Intolerances can also be transient, meaning the person may be able to tolerate the food at a later date.

Food allergy

A food allergy occurs when the body's immune system recognizes a food as harmful and reacts to it. There are three different types of food allergy.

- *IgE-mediated food allergy* This is the most common type of food allergy and one that can cause anaphylaxis (see below). It occurs when the body produces an antibody called immunoglobulin E (IgE) and symptoms develop within minutes or even seconds of eating the food. Sometimes just a trace of that food can cause a reaction, which is why you may hear an announcement that no one can eat peanuts on a plane. In severe cases just a few tiny particles of peanut could induce an anaphylactic reaction.
- *Non-IgE-mediated food allergy* This is when the immune system reacts to a certain food not by producing IgE, but by producing other cells in the immune system. This type of allergy tends to develop more slowly so symptoms may not occur for several hours after ingesting the food.
- *Mixed IgE- and non-IgE-mediated food allergy* This, as the name suggests, is a mixed reaction so symptoms may develop over a wide time frame.

What are the symptoms of a food allergy?

Common symptoms of a food allergy include itching and a rash, like nettle rash, called hives or urticaria. In severe reactions, the face, eyes tongue and lips swell and the person may feel sick and wheezy.

What is anaphylaxis?

An anaphylactic reaction is a severe, life-threatening IgE-mediated allergy. The reaction starts very quickly after ingesting the food and within minutes or seconds the person will notice swelling of the mouth, tongue and lips. They develop difficulty breathing and may feel very lightheaded and collapse. This is a medical emergency and you will need to dial 999 immediately. People who are known to have had an anaphylactic reaction will be offered tests with a specialist to identify the food that caused the reaction and they will be offered an adrenalin pen to carry at all times in case they should come into contact with that food inadvertently.

What foods cause allergies?

Any food can cause an allergic reaction but the common ones are shown below. These foods are different in children and in adults. Children with eczema are more likely to have a food allergy and the more severe the eczema, or the earlier the eczema started, the more likely they are to develop a food allergy. Common triggers include milk, eggs, fish, shellfish, peanuts and tree nuts such as almonds, brazil nuts, walnuts and pistachios. Children often grow out of milk and egg allergies so these are seen much less commonly in adults who are more likely to have an allergy to nuts, fish and shellfish.

What is oral allergy syndrome?

Oral allergy syndrome is usually triggered by eating fresh fruit and vegetables and it presents as itching in the mouth or throat. It is caused by the immune system mistaking proteins on the food as pollens so reacting as you would with hay fever. It is therefore not a true food allergy.

Why can my child eat cakes made with eggs but reacts badly to mayonnaise made with raw eggs?

It is thought that the cooking process may make eggs less allergenic so some children can tolerate eggs if they are well cooked in, for example, a cake but raw eggs in mayonnaise trigger a reaction. The opposite can also be true of some foods. Celery and celeriac, for example, seem to be more allergenic when cooked.

Can I be tested for a food allergy?

You can arrange for blood tests to look for IgE antibodies to any suspected allergenic foods and these will be positive if you have an IgE-mediated food allergy. There are commercially available tests which look for IgG antibodies but, unfortunately, these are not reliable. It is possible to have high levels of IgG in response to common foods and it is thought that this can be a normal reaction rather than an allergic one.

4

Diagnosing irritable
bowel syndrome

Unlike many other bowel conditions IBS is a disorder of bowel function, which means that static pictures of the bowel in the form of X-rays or scans, or even a direct view in the form of a sigmoidoscopy or colonoscopy, will appear normal. Similarly, although you may feel dreadful, your blood tests will be normal. In fact sometimes IBS is diagnosed after extensive testing which has drawn a blank. That is time consuming and expensive and in many cases, with some careful questioning, we can bypass the need for lots of tests.

If you think you may have IBS try to think about how your symptoms affect you and what seems to make them better or worse. It's a good idea to keep a symptom and food diary for at least a couple of weeks. Note down everything you eat and the timing and description of your symptoms. Remember that, as with a food intolerance, there may be a delay of several hours or possibly even days between eating a food and developing symptoms. We all lead busy lives and until it is written down it can be surprisingly difficult to notice a link. Try to score your stress levels too as stress exacerbates IBS symptoms. There is a strong link here – I often see people who are stressed and develop IBS symptoms, they then worry about what could be wrong with them and the more they worry the worse things become, which understandably leaves them convinced something sinister may be going on, meaning yet more worry. It is easy to see how this can become a vicious cycle and managing stress is an important part of managing IBS, which I will cover in Chapter 5.

Women should also take note of their menstrual cycles, as IBS can often flare up in response to hormonal changes around the time of their periods. If you can give an accurate history of your symptoms and what triggers them, your GP will be fairly confident about the diagnosis without needing to examine your abdomen, although we go on to perform an examination to confirm our thoughts. Don't be surprised if your doctor starts by looking at your eyes and hands and feeling in your neck. This will all be normal if you have IBS but your doctor is looking for signs of anaemia or changes in the nail folds that could indicate inflammation in the bowel. Your doctor will want to feel your tummy and may notice any distension and generalized tenderness. He or she may also need to do a rectal examination.

What tests will my doctor do?

There are several tests we can arrange to check your large bowel but if the story is clear cut, they will not be necessary. If there is any doubt, your doctor may arrange any of the following.

Blood tests

There are several blood tests that can be done to check the health of your gastrointestinal system. This doesn't mean several needles though. Your doctor may do some blood tests there and then but he is more likely to ask you to rebook with the practice nurse. The nurse will place a tourniquet around your upper arm and tighten it to occlude the veins and make them swell so that they are easier to see. The nurse may ask you to open and close your fist, which also helps dilate the veins. He or she will then use an alcohol wipe to clean the skin. The most common place to take blood from is the inside of the elbow, at a place called the antecubital fossa. The nurse will use a sterile needle to puncture the vein and collect blood samples into different bottles depending which tests are being done. This shouldn't be painful, but if you are frightened of needles we can use an anaesthetic cream on the skin for 20–30 minutes before the test to numb the skin. If your doctor suggests this, it is worth putting the cream on the inner aspects of both elbows and on the backs of both hands so that there are plenty of options if the veins are difficult to see. Your doctor may want to do tests to check for inflammation, anaemia (IBS shouldn't cause anaemia), and to rule out coeliac disease.

Stool samples

There are two main reasons we arrange stool samples. One is to check for infection and, if your symptoms are predominantly of diarrhoea, your GP may do this to rule out infection. Your doctor will ask you to collect a sample of faeces into a small tube for analysis under a microscope, looking for microorganisms that cause food poisoning and gastroenteritis. The sample is also cultured in a laboratory to see if bugs can be grown so it can take some time for the results to come back. The other reason is to look for microscopic traces of blood in the stool. In this instance, you will be given three stool sample pots and be asked to collect samples from your faeces on three separate occasions and, preferably, from different areas of the stool. These are then sent to the lab to look for traces of blood. If blood is present this is not simply IBS. There could be inflammation, a polyp or even a cancer in the gastrointestinal tract so your doctor will want to arrange further tests to look into this.

Sigmoidoscopy

A sigmoidoscopy involves inserting a long instrument into the anus. This is either a rigid tube about 25 cm long (called a rigid sigmoidoscopy) or a flexible tube about 60 cm long (flexible sigmoidoscopy). Rigid sigmoidoscopy can be performed without bowel preparation but flexible sigmoidoscopy requires the patient to take laxatives before the procedure to clear out the bowel and allow for a better view. Once the instrument is inserted into the anus, rectum and beyond, air is pumped into the sigmoid colon and the doctor can see the lining of this part of the colon under direct vision. In people suffering with irritable bowel syndrome, the passing of this air can reproduce the pain that they experience and, while this is not a diagnostic test, it can help confirm the diagnosis.

Colonoscopy

This is a more invasive procedure, which requires more preparation. You would be asked not to eat and to drink only clear fluids for 24 hours before a colonoscopy and your doctor will give you sachets of a strong laxative to take to ensure that the bowel is empty. You will be given a sedative to have the procedure, which will take 15–30 minutes, during which the doctor will hope to examine your colon all the way up to your caecum or ileum. If you are due to have this procedure make sure that you arrange to be taken to and collected from the hospital, as you will be unable to drive after the sedation.

X-rays

Abdominal X-rays can show constipation, which can be a problem for lots of IBS sufferers.

5

Managing your irritable bowel syndrome

Irritable bowel syndrome is a very individual condition and the first step to managing your IBS is understanding it. Your experience of IBS may be very different to the next person and you may be aware that your own symptoms can fluctuate significantly. I have mentioned food and symptom diaries before and I think they are key to understanding how IBS affects you. Some of my patients, for example, find they can normally get away with certain foodstuffs but if they are stressed, those very foods may trigger symptoms.

There is no doubt that stress and hormones can affect IBS so to get the most from your diary try to write down everything you eat, even the snacks. Take a note of your symptoms, your stress levels and, if you are a woman, your menstrual cycle. Sometimes we lead such busy lives that it is only when things are written down that a pattern begins to emerge. It may not be immediately obvious if there is a link between eating a particular food and developing symptoms as there can be a delay of several hours or even days but if you have kept a clear record, you will be able to look back at your bad days. You can then look at what you ate and how you felt on the days running up to that and gradually you will be able to identify your IBS triggers.

I think of managing IBS under four headings:

- diet
- exercise
- stress
- medication.

Diet for IBS

Managing your diet, if you have IBS, is a bit like the perfect little black dress or a really well fitting suit – what suits one woman or man beautifully just doesn't work for another, which is why the diary is so helpful. If you have IBS it is important that you find time to relax and that you eat regularly. Avoiding meals and leaving long gaps between meals may lead to a flare up of symptoms. Everyone's IBS is different but there are some common triggers that I should mention here and these include:

- alcohol
- caffeine
- fizzy drinks
- fried or fatty food
- processed food.

If you have IBS it is worth monitoring your intake of these foods.

Alcohol Recommended limits for alcohol are just 14 units a week for women and 21 for men and, I'm afraid I am going to frighten you now, that is significantly less than you think. We used to refer to a unit as a small glass of wine, half a pint of beer or a single measure of spirit but as beers and wines have become stronger we need to rethink this. The simple way to calculate your alcohol intake is by looking at the percentage alcohol in the drink you are drinking. The percentage alcohol shows you the number of units in a litre of that drink; so, for wine, a 75 cl bottle is three-quarters of a litre (75 cl = 750 ml; 1 litre = 1000 ml), so if the wine contains 12 per cent alcohol, the number of units in the bottle is three-quarters of 12 = 9 units. If you are pouring a glass at home it is likely to be a 250 ml glass and that will contain 3 units not 1. Alcohol can speed up transit time in the gut, so if you struggle with diarrhoea, it is worth cutting right back on your alcohol intake and some people find it better to cut it out altogether.

Caffeine Similarly, caffeine can stimulate gut activity, making you more prone to diarrhoea. If this is you, try to limit your intake to three cups of tea or coffee a day. Try decaffeinated varieties, although be careful, as even decaffeinated drinks often contain some caffeine and you may prefer to opt for herbal teas as a replacement.

Fizzy drinks If bloating and flatulence are a problem to you, cutting back on fizzy drinks may help alleviate your symptoms.

Fried or fatty food Fatty foods can be more difficult to digest, leading to diarrhoea, so reducing your intake of these may help reduce symptoms. This means cutting back on cakes, biscuits, chocolate and pastries. Try to use sprays rather than spreads for cooking and opt for low-fat sauces and dressings. Wherever possible try to boil, steam, grill or poach your food rather than fry it. Try to limit your saturated fat intake from butter, cheese, meat, cakes and pastries and swap these for unsaturated fats found in vegetable oils, nuts and seeds.

Processed food Processed foods tend to contain resistant starches, which are more difficult to digest, meaning they arrive in the large colon undigested. They are then fermented by the gut flora resulting in the production of wind, meaning bloating and flatulence. Cutting back on the amount of processed food you eat will improve these symptoms.

What about fibre?

When I was at medical school we were taught that people with IBS should increase their fibre intake, but in fact not all fibre is the same. When we think of fibre we need to think of it in terms of soluble and insoluble fibre. If you are trying to increase your total fibre intake, try to increase your soluble fibre not your insoluble fibre.

- *Soluble fibre* By soluble fibre we mean fibre that dissolves in water and can be broken down by gut bacteria. Soluble fibre helps to keep stools soft and can be found in oats, barley, rye, nuts, seeds, fruit, vegetables, beans and pulses.
- *Insoluble fibre* Insoluble fibre does not dissolve in water and so passes intact through the gut and allows waste to pass through the bowel more quickly. It is found in wholegrains, bran, corn, wheat and nuts. Cutting back on these foods may help if diarrhoea is a problem to you.

Linseed is a source of both soluble and insoluble fibre. A tablespoon a day added to meals may help ease the symptoms of IBS, but beware of increasing your fibre intake too quickly as this may make symptoms of bloating and flatulence temporarily worse.

Fructose

Fructose is a naturally occurring sugar in fruit. It is actually not very well absorbed in the body and can predispose to diarrhoea. It is recommended that we all eat at least five portions of fruit and vegetables a day but, if you are struggling with diarrhoea, it may be worth limiting your fruit intake and making up the rest with vegetables. You may have also heard of the term 'high-fructose corn syrup'. This is used in a lot of processed foods so get into the habit of checking food labels and keep your intake of this to a minimum.

- *Artificial sweeteners* Artificial sweeteners containing sorbitol have a laxative effect so beware your intake of these.
- *Fluids* The standard advice is to drink 8–10 cups of water a day but, to be honest, it is total fluid intake that is important. Herbal teas and weak squashes are fine and I don't get too hung up on absolute volumes because it depends on ambient temperature and how active you are. The simplest way to know if you are drinking enough is to check the colour of your urine. It should be straw coloured. If it is darker than that then you need to increase your fluid intake.

What about probiotics?

The theory behind adding a daily probiotic to your diet is to top up the good bacteria in your gut and aid digestion. They don't work for everyone but some of my patients report a significant improvement in the symptoms of bloating and diarrhoea when they take a daily probiotic. Different brands contain different mixtures of good bacteria, so if after four weeks you don't feel any difference, it is worth trying an alternative brand. Products containing *Bifidobacterium lactis* can help with bloating and abdominal pain.

Dr Dawn's top tips

If you are considering making changes to your diet to help your IBS, remember this:

- be patient – it can take a few weeks for things to improve;
- try to eat regularly;
- sit down to eat and allow yourself time to digest your food.

Exercise for IBS

Sadly, fewer than a third of UK adults exercise to recommended levels. If constipation is a problem to you with your IBS, then increasing your activity level will help. That doesn't have to mean joining a fancy gym; in fact if you hate the gym, it doesn't matter how smart the facilities look or how many of your friends are raving about the place. If you don't like exercising in a gym, then you may force yourself to stick with it for a small number of weeks, maybe even a small number of months but, as sure as eggs are eggs, you won't be doing it this time next year. And exercise is like healthy eating. You need to make small changes that, hand on heart, you think you will be able to keep up for good. I know this because, over the years, I have joined gyms. I join in January and, by spring, I have usually fallen by the wayside – and that's because I get bored in a gym.

A few years ago I was run over by a car and shattered my left knee. Part of my rehabilitation was sitting on a static bicycle in a physiotherapy gym, trying to flex my knee enough to do a single revolution. When I achieved this, I was so desperate to build the strength up in my damaged leg and regain full mobility that I started cycling in the lanes near my house. I found that this was something I really enjoyed. Ten minutes on a bike in the gym and I'm clock watching but cycling in the countryside just ticked boxes for me and I started cycling with friends in the village. I have always been a great believer in exercising with friends because when your motivation is low they will spur you on, and you will do the same for them. Before I knew it, I had signed up to a charity ride from London to Paris – and that ticked another box. There is nothing like the fear of failure to make sure you get out and train whatever your motivation or the weather outside. So I learned a lot about myself: I prefer exercising outside; I need friends to force me out when I'm feeling lazy; and I need a challenge to make me stick to my training schedule. The boxes you need to tick may be completely different. Just feeling physically better as your bowels become more regular may be all the motivation you need.

We recommend that everyone walks at least 10,000 paces a day and, ideally, that should be your baseline with formal exercise on top of that. The average pace is 50–75 cm long which means, if you achieve your 10,000 steps, you will walk 5–7.5 km in a day just going about your business! A while back I decided to practise what I preach and invested in a pedometer. I think of myself as quite an active person and certainly at weekends I had no problem clocking in my 10,000 paces. Busy days in surgery were a totally different matter, and I found that sitting at my desk calling in patients meant it was easy to get to 6.30 p.m. and be frighteningly short of my target. I decided then to get up and walk to the waiting room rather than use an intercom calling system. It meant I could maintain my activity levels on my surgery days and I actually prefer it. It is so much more personal than calling people through using a tannoy. This simple change meant I was staying on target and, in this day of internet technology, emails, texts and all the other ways of communicating with the outside world without actually moving, it can be all too easy to get to the end of your day without having moved much at all. If you're not moving, the chances are your bowels may not either!

It doesn't matter what you do, but if your job is sedentary you will have to make a definite decision to move more. Maybe you get off the bus or the tube a stop early? Maybe you use the stairs instead of an escalator or a lift? Maybe you promise yourself that you will walk over to your colleague's desk to discuss an issue rather than just press 'send' on an email? Whatever you decide to do, invest in a pedometer and start counting your daily steps. This is what I call baseline activity. Once you have achieved this, you need to think about exercise on top and, ideally, you should be aiming for 30 minutes a day at least five times a week. It doesn't matter what it is but you need to get a bit short of breath doing it. The sort of shortness of breath that means you talk in short phrases and need to catch your breath. If you are gasping for air you are overdoing it and need to take the pressure off, but if you are chatting happily then don't kid yourself – you may be keeping active but you are not truly exercising in my book and you need to push yourself a bit harder!

If you want to get a little more technical, buy yourself a heart rate monitor to wear while you are exercising. When you are fit, you should aim for a pulse rate between 70 and 85 per cent of your maximum heart rate (MHR). If you are just starting out 60 per cent of your MHR is probably more realistic. You can calculate your MHR by subtracting your age from 220 if you are a man, or 210 if you are a woman. So, if you are a man aged 40, your MHR is:

220 – 40 = 180.

Your optimum training range is 70–85 per cent of 180, which is:

70% of 180 = (70 ÷ 100) × 180 = 126 beats per minute
85% of 180 = (85 ÷ 100) × 180 = 153 beats per minute.

Stress and IBS

We all respond to stress differently and what one person finds unacceptable, another can tolerate perfectly well, and some stress can be good for us. It makes us feel more alert and focused. There is a fine line though and ignoring the signs of stress on a day to day basis can have a detrimental effect on our health. The problem is that, evolutionarily, we have not adapted to modern day stresses as well as we might. If your stress comes in the form of a mammoth, it is completely appropriate that you are firing on adrenalin and ready to run, or to stand and fight your ground – the classic 'fight or flight' reaction. The problem is that today's stresses don't come in the form of the occasional mammoth, they come in the form of deadlines and juggling home and work and relationship problems.

If you have IBS, you will almost certainly recognize that your symptoms flare up when you are under pressure. Of course there may be some stresses you can do nothing about, but with a little forward planning you may be able to juggle your diary to keep stress at a manageable level. I will discuss medication next but I have lots of patients who use medication on an occasional basis. If they know they are about to hit a tough time at work or if things are difficult at home, they start medication to cover them through that time and that is completely appropriate. The other thing to say here is that it is OK to factor in a bit of down time! It is so easy to feel guilty about booking in a massage or a session of acupuncture but that's exactly the sort of thing that may help and, believe me, you will be a better work colleague, better partner, better friend and better parent if you feel comfortable and have your IBS under control. If stress is a real problem to you, it may be that one of the talking therapies such as cognitive behavioural therapy is something to consider and your GP will be able to advise about local services.

Medication and IBS

Many people with IBS will be able to manage their symptoms with the lifestyle changes mentioned above but others will need medication and, as I have already intimated, some people will take medication on a regular basis while others will use it when their symptoms flare up and may then have a period when they don't need it.

There are four main classes of pills that I use in treating IBS and these include:

- anti-spasmodics
- laxatives
- anti-diarrhoeals
- anti-depressants.

Anti-spasmodics

These work by relaxing the muscle in the bowel wall. Some are available over the counter from your pharmacist and others need a prescription from your GP. They include hyoscine, mebeverine and alverine. Peppermint oil taken in capsule form also relaxes the bowel wall but can cause heartburn. Most pharmacies today have private consultation rooms where you can discuss your symptoms confidentially. Make sure you know exactly how you should take the medication as some need to be taken 20–30 minutes before a meal.

Laxatives

There are different forms of laxative and again your pharmacist will be able to advise. We tend to recommend bulk-forming laxatives for IBS sufferers and you will need to allow a few days for them to work before gradually increasing the dose. I sometimes use osmotic laxatives in IBS too but stimulant laxatives can make cramping pains worse and, if used too regularly, the bowel can become acclimatized to them:

- *Bulking agents*, such as ispaghula husk or methylcellulose. These are basically sources of extra fibre and work by bulking out the stool. They take a few days to work.
- *Osmotic laxatives*, such as lactulose and the macrogols. These work by increasing the amount of fluid in the motion, so softening the stool. Again they can take several days to work.
- *Stimulant laxatives*, such as senna or bisocodyl. These work by stimulating the muscle in the bowel wall and should work overnight. They shouldn't be used long term as the bowel can start to rely on them.

Anti-diarrhoeals

An anti-diarrhoeal, such as loperamide, works by slowing down the muscle in the bowel wall, meaning that food takes longer to travel along the gut allowing more time for absorption.

Anti-depressants

There are two main types of anti-depressants that I use to treat IBS I use them in people who have been unable to control their symptoms with the measures above and they can be amazingly effective. They include an old-fashioned class of drugs called the tricyclic anti-depressants. I tend to use these in low doses as a first line, as I have seen such great results. As a second choice I sometimes try newer selective serotonin re-uptake inhibitors.

6
FAQs

Is IBS a lifelong condition?

About 20 per cent of the population have IBS at any one time but actually around one in ten sufferers each year will notice their symptoms have subsided. It isn't a condition that we cure as such but just because your symptoms are interfering with your life now, that doesn't mean it will always be so. Most people notice periods when their symptoms improve for weeks, months or even years and some find their symptoms disappear completely.

Are there any long-term complications of IBS?

People often worry about a possible link between IBS and bowel cancer, for example, but there is no evidence that there is any link here. Sometimes I meet people who have developed depression as a result of their IBS but that is because they have been really dragged down by symptoms and, hopefully, after reading this book you won't be one of them!

Is lactose intolerance linked to IBS?

Lactose intolerance and IBS are separate conditions. One doesn't cause the other but it is possible to have the two conditions at the same time.

Can IBS cause rectal bleeding?

IBS can cause constipation which in turn can cause haemorrhoids or an anal fissure (a tear in the delicate skin around the anus). Both of these can cause fresh rectal bleeding but IBS itself does not so blood in the stools should always be checked out by a doctor. It is usually something simple like piles or a tear but bleeding from the back passage can be caused by a cancer so should never be ignored.

What is post-infectious IBS?

Post-infectious IBS was first described after the Second World War when soldiers were returning from war having had bacterial dysentery. It has since become a well-recognized condition and has been described following infections with campylobacter, salmonella and shigella. Interestingly, it is uncommon after viral gut infections and generally occurs after a bacterial infection. The good news is that 50 per cent of people recover without the need for treatment.

7

The low-FODMAP diet

FODMAP stands for Fermentable Oligosaccharides, Disaccharides, Monosaccharides and Polyols. These are carbohydrates that are not well absorbed in the small gut so arrive in the large gut to be broken down by the bacteria in the colon, in a process called fermentation, which produces gas as a by-product. This also means that more fluid enters the large bowel, which can lead to diarrhoea. The low-FODMAP diet is a relatively new and complex diet, which works on the theory that if you reduce your intake of these carbohydrates, you will reduce the amount of gas production and therefore improve the symptoms of bloating. The diet was originally developed in Melbourne, Australia, and has been adapted here in the UK by researchers at King's College in London. It is generally reserved for those IBS sufferers who have been unable to control their IBS symptoms with the measures described in Chapter 5. It is a complex diet and if you are considering trying it, you will need the help of a qualified dietician. In essence, you need to cut out FODMAP foods for a period of four to eight weeks, which is a long time and will take a degree of dedication. After this period you will be advised how to gradually reintroduce foods. The whole concept is that no two IBS sufferers are the same, as I have said before; this is a very individual condition and your dietician will be able to advise you so that you can work out your own levels of tolerance to different foods and combinations of foods.

The researchers at King's College, London say that this diet works for about 76 per cent of IBS sufferers. It targets the bowel symptoms and has not yet been shown to improve other associated symptoms, such as headaches and fatigue. High-FODMAP foods include those foods containing:

- *fructose*, found in fruits such as apples and pears;
- *fructan*, found in onions, wheat, artichokes and asparagus;

- *raffinose*, found in cabbage and lentils;
- *sorbitol*, found in plums and artificial sweeteners.]

You'll find more information on the low-FODMAP diet in the FODMAP-friendly recipes section below.

8

FODMAP-friendly recipes

Disclaimer

Please note that research on FODMAP foods is ongoing and the advice given here may change as FODMAP research advances. The ideas within this book are intended only as a guide. Manufacturers do alter ingredients so it is important to check product ingredient lists to ensure foods and drinks are FODMAP friendly. Following the low-FODMAP diet is not recommended without specialist dietary advice from a registered dietitian. Your chances of success are reduced if you don't follow the low-FODMAP diet effectively.

Additional serving size recommendations for fruit and veg can be found on the Monash University low FODMAP diet app at <www.med.monash.edu.au/cecs/gastro/FODMAP/iphone-app.html>.

If you think leading a low-FODMAP lifestyle means the end to flavoursome food, then think again. With a few adjustments, you can still enjoy family favourites like spaghetti Bolognese and chilli con carne, Italian-style risottos, hearty soups, stir-fries, roast chicken and more. Baking isn't off limits either. Simply ensure you have the suitable ingredients to hand.

Most of these delicious recipes use quick and easy short cuts, such as bought stock pots, canned or frozen vegetables, and steamed rice pouches. You can team up any meal with a FODMAP-friendly side salad, and most of the dishes can be stored and enjoyed the next day if you have any leftovers. As well as the ideas within this book, you'll find a range of websites that provide free access to lots of other healthy and tasty low-FODMAP recipes.

Table 1 Your quick guide to FODMAPs

FODMAP stands for		Type of carbohydrate	Found in these foods*
F	Fermentable		
O	Oligosaccharides:	fructans	wheat, rye, barley, onion, garlic, inulin
		GOS (galactooligosaccharides)	all beans and pulses, cashew, pistachio nuts
D	Disaccharides:	lactose	cow's, sheep's and goat's milk and yoghurts, soft cheeses e.g. cottage cheese
M	Monosaccharides:	fructose	honey, mango, apples, pears, asparagus, fructose sugars/syrups, fruit juices
A	and		
P	Polyols:	sorbitol	stone fruits and sugar-free chewing gum and mints
		mannitol	mushrooms and cauliflower
		xylitol	sugar-free chewing gum and mints

*NB: These are not the only foods FODMAP carbohydrates are found in.

Be supermarket savvy

Take note of the following tips that will help you to choose suitable low-FODMAP ingredients for your store cupboard.

Ready meals and shop-bought soups

Sometimes you just haven't got the time to cook, and so short cuts from the supermarket can get very tempting. But ready meals and packet or canned soups will almost certainly contain onion or garlic, and so are best avoided for your 4–8-week low-FODMAP elimination trial. The meal ideas provided below aim to provide you with quick and tasty FODMAP-friendly home-cooked meals and snacks.

Gravy, stock and sauces

The majority of these contain FODMAP ingredients such as onion, dried onion powder, garlic and garlic powder. At the time of printing, Knorr Flavour Pots can be a useful store cupboard addition: Paprika, Curry, Garden Herbs, Mixed Herbs, Mixed Chilli and 3 Peppercorn are all suitable flavours.

Onion and garlic alternatives

If you need flavour minus the FODMAPs, try garlic-, basil- or chilli-infused oils, finely sliced spring onions (green stems only), finely sliced leek leaves (green part only), dried or fresh chives, and asafoetida 'hing' powder for a FODMAP-friendly flavour hit.

Salad ideas

Choose any of the following ingredients to create your colourful crispy salad base: fresh tomato (a medium tomato counts as 1 fruit serving); sliced green stems of spring onion; sliced red, yellow, orange or green pepper; celery (use ¼ of a stick); grated carrot; cucumber slices; sweetcorn (use less than 3 tbsp); 2 slices of beetroot; bean sprouts and radishes. For salad leaves, try iceberg, endive, red coral, radicchio, butter lettuce, rocket, baby spinach, or chard.

Low-FODMAP foods shopping list

Planning your shopping in advance will really help you to get started on your 4–8-week low-FODMAP elimination diet.

Tips to help you complete your shopping list

- Using the meal ideas provided below, plan your meals for the week or days ahead. Have a look at the breakfast, lunch and evening meal ideas and highlight what you will need on the starter shopping list. Note that is a guide only. For more details on portion sizes, check out the Monash app mentioned in the Disclaimer at the start of this chapter.
- If you know that you will need some snacks, include some healthy choices on your shopping list rather than trying to find them at the last minute.

FODMAP-friendly grains and starchy carbs

- 'Gluten-free' or 'free from' breads, rolls, pitta, wraps, bagels, crumpets, crackers and cereals
- Rice Krispies or gluten-free cornflakes
- Rice cakes, plain
- Corn taco shells
- Gluten-free self-raising or plain flours (if baking)
- Cornflour, if making gravy or as a sauce/soup thickener
- 'Free from' pasta
- All varieties of rice (white or brown)
- Quinoa
- Buckwheat
- Polenta
- Plain oats (limit to 25 g / 1 sachet per serving)
- Oat or rice bran
- Approximately four oat cakes per serving
- Potatoes
- Rice noodles or 100 per cent buckwheat soba noodles e.g. Amoy 'Straight to Wok' rice noodles.

Note that you need to double-check that no unsuitable FODMAP ingredients have been added to shop-bought breads, cereals or crackers; for example, apple juice, honey, inulin, FOS or fruit juice concentrate.

Meat, fish, eggs, pulses, nuts, seeds

- Lean, cooked red meats: beef, lamb, pork
- Chicken and turkey
- Lean minced beef, lamb or turkey or Quorn mince
- Roast joint of your choice
- Corned beef
- Canned or fresh oily fish e.g. mackerel, sardines, salmon, tuna
- Fillet of white fish e.g. haddock, plaice
- Shellfish e.g. prawns, scallops
- Nuts (but avoid cashew nuts and pistachios)
- Seeds of choice
- Canned chickpeas
- Canned lentils

- Red split lentils, boiled
- Quorn chicken pieces
- Peanut butter
- Eggs
- Plain tofu or tempeh
- Dairy and dairy-free alternatives
- Milks:
    - lactose-free milk e.g. Arla's 'Lacto-free'
    - calcium-enriched dairy-free milks e.g. soya (from hulled beans only; avoid milk made from whole soya beans), coconut, almond, rice or oat milks.

Cheeses

- Hard or semi-ripe cheeses e.g. Cheddar, Brie, Parmesan, feta, goats cheese, halloumi
- Pre-grated mozzarella or, if you prefer, one small packet (150 g) of milky mozzarella
- Cottage cheese, ricotta – up to 2 tbsp per serving
- Lactose-free cream cheese e.g. Philadelphia.

Yoghurts and dessert toppers

Generally up to 2 tbsp per serving of a plain or a FODMAP-friendly fruit yoghurt is well tolerated e.g. as a muesli/granola/fruit salad topper.

- Lactose-free yoghurts – only available in strawberry or raspberry
- Soya yoghurts e.g. Alpro Big Pot: plain, plain with coconut, plain with almond or strawberry and rhubarb
- Low-lactose ice cream or up to one scoop of FODMAP-friendly dairy milk ice cream
- Swedish Glaze soya ice cream
- Whipped cream
- Alpro soya custard or up to 2 tbsp normal custard.

Note, again, that you need to double-check that no unsuitable FODMAP ingredients have been added to shop-bought breads, cereals or crackers; for example, apple juice, honey, inulin, FOS or fruit juice concentrate.

Fruit

Limit fruit to three servings spaced throughout the day.

- FODMAP-friendly pure juice e.g. orange, pineapple, grape juice (limit to one small glass 100 ml/day)
- Banana or banana chips
- Berries e.g. strawberries, blueberries, raspberries
- Dried cranberries, dried coconut, currants, raisins – less than 1 tbsp per serving
- Kiwi, melon (cantaloupe and honeydew)
- Oranges, clementines, mandarins
- All grapes
- Grapefruit
- Lemons and limes
- Pineapple (avoid dried), passion fruit, pomegranate seeds
- Rhubarb.

Vegetables and salad

- Aubergine, broccoli, butternut squash
- Courgettes, carrots, celeriac, chilli, celery, chives, half a corn on the cob
- Green beans, ginger root, kale, leek (green leaves only)
- Pumpkin, parsnips, peas
- Stir-fry: bok choy/pak choi, bamboo shoots, bean sprouts, water chestnuts
- Salad items: 4 cherry or 1 tomato (count as 1 fruit serving), cucumber, spring onions (green part only), pepper, radish, baby spinach, rocket leaves, Swiss chard, sweetcorn
- Turnip
- White cabbage.

Fats and sugars

Check your store cupboard's jam/marmalade ingredients as you may need to purchase a different brand; unsuitable FODMAP ingredients commonly found in these include e.g. fructose, glucose-fructose syrup, apple juice concentrate or other unsuitable fruits.

- FODMAP-friendly jam and marmalades
- Regular table sugar

- Maple syrup, golden syrup
- Any vegetable oil e.g. olive or rapeseed oils, garlic-, basil- or chilli-infused oils
- Butter or margarine of choice.

Snacks

When shopping for snacks choose products that do not contain unsuitable FODMAP ingredients e.g. fructose, inulin, apple juice concentrate, honey, agave nectar.

- FODMAP-friendly mixed nuts and seeds – you could add small handful of FODMAP-friendly dried fruit and make your own trail mix (a small handful of dried coconut is suitable too)
- Olives – plain or with herbs/chilli/feta pieces
- Dark chocolate or 50 g milk or white, chocolate coated rice cakes, sesame snap bars
- 9Bar: peanut or cracked pepper
- 9Bar Indulgence: Cocoa and Raspberry, Cocoa and Coconut, Cocoa and Hazelnut
- FODMAP-friendly 'gluten-free/free from' biscuits/cakes
- Plain or salt and vinegar potato crisps, plain pretzels
- Homemade or shop-bought popcorn (check ingredients)
- Homemade FODMAP-friendly oat cookie, scone or pancake from recipe ideas provided in this chapter.

Condiments and flavourings

- Tomato sauce, tartare sauce, mint sauce, mustard, mayonnaise and salad cream
- Compton's gravy salt, Maggi beef stock cube or stock pot
- Knorr low-salt chicken stock cube or granules, Maggi chicken stock cube or stock pot
- Vegetable stock cubes are often unsuitable. You can make your own vegetable stock with FODMAP-friendly veg or All New Knorr Flavour Pots (not garlic) are a great alternative
- Asafoetida 'hing' powder
- Worcestershire sauce, BBQ sauce, sweet and sour sauce, soy sauce, fish sauce and oyster sauce, Tabasco
- All vinegars including cider, balsamic (less than 1 tbsp), red and white wine

- Tomato purée or plain passata sauce
- Tinned tomatoes, plain or with added herbs e.g. basil (½ a tin = 1 tomato/fruit serving).

Check the ingredient lists in the condiments, stocks and gravy in your store cupboard. You may need to purchase a different brand; unsuitable FODMAP ingredients commonly found in these items include e.g. fructose, onion, garlic, wheat, barley.

Low-FODMAP baking tips

Gluten-free (GF) recipes are a useful place to start. We know flours made from rice, potatoes, quinoa, corn (maize), buck-wheat, sorghum, and teff are gluten-free and have also tested low for FODMAPs. But, gluten-free recipes are becoming increasingly adventurous and often use a wide variety of different GF flours, seeds, tubers and beans such as oats, amaranth, soya bean, chickpea (garbanzo), and fava (broad) beans. Although these are gluten-free, they have all tested amber or red for FODMAPs by the Monash University team in Australia. People may find they have to avoid or limit foods made from these flours to suit their individual tolerance levels. The low-FODMAP diet app by the Monash team provides more information on suitable FODMAP-friendly serving sizes of these GF foods.

In the UK, there is a huge variety of individual gluten-free flours available in supermarkets, health food shops and online. Popular FODMAP-friendly, 'All purpose' GF flours include Dove's Farm and Glebe Farm. These are made from a blend of rice, corn and potato starch. The Dove's Farm blend also contains tapioca, which is not yet tested for FODMAPs.

Remember that when you use online gluten-free recipes, you will need to check that all the additional ingredients in the recipe are also suitable for a low-FODMAP diet. Many recipes may call for honey, high-FODMAP fruit and vegetables, onion, garlic and so on, so you'll need to make suitable swaps where necessary.

A note on xanthan gum

This is a natural gluten-free starch produced by fermentation. It is widely used in foods as a thickener and will appear in ingredients lists as xanthan gum or E415.

Xanthan gum is a useful ingredient for gluten-free baking, as it helps to improve the texture of your baking, whether it's bread, cakes or pastry, as it works in a similar way to gluten. Xanthan gum comes in a powder and you can add it to recipes as suggested. You may find you need to add a little more liquid than stated in the recipes, as xanthan gum thickens quite a lot. You can find xanthan gum in the 'free from' aisle of some of the major supermarkets and health food shops.

Breakfast ideas

Breakfast really is an important part of your daily routine. Research shows that breakfast eaters are better able to keep to a healthy weight. Dieters tend to go short on B vitamins, so if you can, try to get yours from low-FODMAP fortified breakfast cereal (such as cornflakes or Rice Krispies). If you like, you can add a little oat or rice bran to your cereal for extra fibre. Gluten-free bread is usually low in fibre, but a slice of spelt bread typically contains just as much fibre as wholemeal bread. Weight for weight, they have the same calories, but because a slice of spelt bread tends to be heavier, each slice will be higher in calories than wholemeal bread. Not eating enough food can mean your immune system is below par, so make sure you get a daily supply of antioxidants by eating your allowance of fruit and vegetables. If you need to keep an eye on your cholesterol levels, choose a heart-healthy breakfast that contains soluble fibre, such as oats in porridge. Oats contain slowly digested carbs and have a low glycaemic index. This, coupled with the protein from the lactose-free milk, can help you feel fuller for longer.

Four FODMAP-friendly breakfast cereal toppers

1 Fresh fruit (limit to an 80 g serving): blueberries, raspberries, strawberries, banana, grapes, slice of honeydew or cantaloupe melon

2 Dried fruit (limit to under 1 tbsp): dried cranberries, raisins, goji berries or banana chips
3 Nuts: pecans, walnuts, peanuts, macadamia, fewer than ten hazelnuts and almonds, Brazil nuts
4 Seeds: pumpkin, sunflower, chia, linseeds and sesame seeds.

Breakfasts in three simple steps

Warm and oaty

1 Take one of these:
   - 25 g of porridge oats, or
   - 1 shop-bought plain sachet of porridge oats, or
   - oat-based breakfast cereal e.g. Oat Flakes;
2 Choose lactose-free milk or FODMAP-friendly calcium-enriched dairy-free alternative;
3 Add a fruit and nut breakfast cereal topper of your choice.

Crispy and crunchy

1 A serving of Rice Krispies or gluten-free cornflakes;
2 Lactose-free milk or FODMAP-friendly calcium-enriched dairy-free alternative;
3 Add a fruit and nut breakfast cereal topper of your choice.

Eggs 'n' 'cherries

1 Boiled, poached or scrambled egg;
2 Serve with toasted FODMAP-friendly 'free from' bread;
3 A side serving of warm cherry tomatoes (count tomatoes as one fruit serving).

Toast topper

1 Toasted FODMAP-friendly 'free from' bread or rice cakes;
2 Top with sliced banana;
3 Throw on some peanut butter.

Berry-licious yoghurt

1 Handful of berries;
2 Top with 3–4 tbsp of *plain* soya yoghurt or a lactose-free flavoured yoghurt;

3 Sprinkle with a handful of FODMAP-friendly nuts or seeds of your choice.

Note that you may find unsuitable fruits, fruit juice concentrates, honey, FOS, inulin, or oligofructose in gluten-free/free from products and dairy-free alternatives such as soya milks and yoghurts. Always double-check ingredients, foods and drinks for these FODMAPs.

Lunch ideas

Lunch needn't be a standard sandwich made from white, crumbly gluten-free bread. Many supermarkets now stock tasty gluten-free breads, some with added calcium, and you can even get gluten-free pitta bread to give your lunchtime a Mediterranean twist. Choose a variety of fillings such as ham, tuna, cheese, egg and salad. Make the most of low-FODMAP veggies by creating a hearty soup that you can take to work on cold winter days, and in the summer you might prefer a fresh, crispy salad with an olive oil and lemon juice dressing. Add some sliced chicken or tuna if you like. If you enjoy being creative in the kitchen, you could also make a gluten-free pizza topped with low-FODMAP vegetables such as aubergine, peppers, courgettes and sweetcorn.

Three tasty steps to lunch

Light 'n' crispy

1 Take a couple of rice cakes or toasted FODMAP-friendly 'free-from' pitta bread;
2 Spread on some crunchy peanut butter and a sliced banana;
3 Finish with a sprinkling of sesame or chia seeds for extra crunch.

Jumbo jacket

1 Large baked potato;
2 Filling of your choice e.g. grated hard cheese and a sliced tomato (count tomato as 1 fruit serving); 2–3 tbsp of sweetcorn mixed with a tablespoon of lactose-free cream cheese and freshly ground black pepper, homemade egg mayonnaise or cottage cheese (max 3 tbsp cottage cheese), homemade low-FODMAP chilli or Bolognese;

3 Serve your potato and chosen filling with a FODMAP-friendly side salad.

Sumptuous soup

1 Homemade soup – see recipes below;
2 Serve with a FODMAP-friendly 'free from' roll or bread, or make them into toasted croutons;
3 Sprinkle with fresh chives.

Wrap it up

1 FODMAP-friendly 'free from' wrap spread with tomato purée (count tomato as 1 fruit serving);
2 Top with canned tuna, or sliced cooked chicken, sprinkle with grated or sliced mozzarella cheese, basil leaves and a few fresh tomato slices;
3 Heat through under a hot grill. Serve with a FODMAP-friendly side salad of choice.

Cheese please

1 Take some Brie or Camembert;
2 Lay slivers on oatcakes;
3 Serve with a handful of grapes.

Omega-3 boost

1 FODMAP-friendly 'free from' crackers;
2 Top with canned oily fish e.g. sardines, mackerel, salmon or 1–2 smoked salmon slices;
3 Serve with a FODMAP-friendly side salad of choice.

FODMAP-friendly soups

Soups can be a lifesaver if you're pushed for time, as most of them freeze quite easily. Prepare them in bulk and freeze in individual containers, so you have a wholesome starter or light meal ready on those busy weeknights. Cook for as long as you like – some people prefer chunky and crispy vegetables in soup, while others like puréed, creamy soups. Mix and match so you get a variety of textures. As well as the traditional hob method, all these soups can also be cooked in a pressure cooker for about 12–15 minutes, then blended.

Carrot and coriander soup

Prep 5 mins. *Cook* 20 mins. *Serves* 6

1 tbsp olive or rapeseed oil

1 tsp ground coriander

4–5 medium sized carrots, peeled and roughly sliced

1 litre of chicken stock (see Box, below)

Large handful of coriander, freshly chopped, if desired

Heat 1 tbsp of olive or rapeseed oil in a large pan, add the ground coriander and cook for approximately 1 min. Add the carrots and the stock, bring to the boil, and then reduce the heat. Cover and cook for 15–20 minutes until the carrots are tender. Blend with a hand blender or tip into a food processor with the coriander and blitz until smooth. Taste and season as required.

Stock cubes

Knorr low-salt chicken cubes or granules are one of the few stocks not to mention onion/garlic in their ingredients list. 'Flavouring' is mentioned in Knorr stock cubes and although there is a possibility that onion is part of this, most people on a low-FODMAP diet do seem to tolerate these well. Maggi chicken cubes and stock pots are also suitable. Check ingredients regularly in case manufacturers have changed the recipe. Where the recipes call for chicken stock, use a Knorr low-salt chicken cube or granules; Maggi chicken cube or stock pot; or a Knorr herb Flavour Pot.

Butternut squash or sweet potato soup

Prep 10 mins. *Cook* 25–30 mins. *Serves* 6

1 tbsp vegetable or chilli-infused oil

1 small butternut squash, peeled, deseeded and sliced OR 1 sweet potato, peeled and sliced

2 carrots, peeled and sliced

Dried chilli flakes, pinch (optional)

1 litre of chicken stock (see Box, page 45)

Handful of chopped fresh flat leaf parsley (or 1 tsp dried) to season before serving, if desired

Heat 1 tbsp of vegetable or chilli-infused oil in a large pan, add the squash or sweet potato and carrots and cook over a medium heat for 3–4 minutes. For an extra chilli kick you could also add a pinch of dried chilli flakes too. Add the stock and bring to the boil. Lower the heat and simmer for 15–20 minutes or until all the vegetables are tender. Remove from heat and allow to cool. Tip into a food processor or use a hand blender. Add the parsley and blitz until smooth. Taste and season as required.

Tomato and basil soup

Prep 10 mins. *Cook* 15 mins. *Serves* 4–6

Basil-infused oil

1 tsp dried oregano

Fresh thyme sprigs or 1 tsp dried thyme

2–3 handfuls of fresh basil leaves or 1 tsp dried basil

Salt and pepper

1 tsp sugar

2 × (400 g) tins peeled tomatoes

400 ml hot chicken stock (see Box, page 45)

200 ml lactose-free milk

Sugar, to taste

Cornflour, to thicken

Heat ½ tbsp of basil-infused oil in a large pan and add the oregano, thyme and basil. Stir and warm the herbs through the oil. Season with salt, pepper and a tsp of sugar. Add the peeled tomatoes with the juice. Pour in the stock and bring to the boil. Reduce the temperature, remove the lid and simmer for about 10 minutes. Remove the soup from hob and allow to cool. Remove the thyme sprigs. Tip into a food processor or use a hand blender. Add the milk and blitz until smooth, thickened with cornflour as required. Taste and season if required with salt, pepper or sugar. Count a bowl as 1 fruit serving.

Roasted red pepper soup

Prep 10 mins. *Cook* 15 mins. *Serves* 2–3

1 red pepper, cored and seeds removed, roughly chopped

Handful of fresh thyme or 1 tsp dried thyme

2 tbsp garlic-infused oil

500 ml of chicken stock (see Box, page 45)

50 ml double cream (optional)

Salt and pepper

Preheat the oven to gas mark 6 / 200°C / 400°F. Place the red pepper, thyme and garlic-infused oil into a bowl and season, to taste, with salt and freshly ground black pepper. Pour onto a clean baking sheet and roast in the oven for approximately 12 minutes, or until tender and cooked. Allow to cool. Transfer the roasted pepper to a food processor. Add the stock and double cream, if using; season well and blend until smooth.

Main meals

Fish noodle supper

Prep 10 mins. *Cook* 15–20 mins. *Serves* 1

Fillet of white fish of your choice, about 150 g

1 tsp chilli-infused oil

Pinch of dried chilli flakes (optional)

1 tsp rapeseed oil

1–2 stir-fry FODMAP-friendly vegetables of choice e.g. green beans

1 packet of 'Straight to Wok' rice noodles or 1 dried nest or 150 g fresh cooked noodles

1 tbsp oyster, soy, or fish sauce to flavour

Preheat the oven to gas mark 5 / 190°C / 375°F. Place the fish on a greased baking tray and drizzle over the chilli-infused oil and a pinch of dried chilli flakes, if desired. Bake for about 15 mins. Meanwhile, heat the rapeseed oil in a wok, add 1–2 stir-fry veg of choice, e.g. sliced green beans (up to 12), and stir-fry for 5–6 minutes. Add 1 packet of 'Straight to Wok' rice noodles and stir-fry for further 3 mins. Stir through 1 tbsp soy, fish or oyster sauce to flavour and pour over the excess chilli juice from the fish. Serve the cooked fish on top of the noodle stir-fry.

Singapore-style prawn noodles

Prep 10 mins. *Cook* 10 mins. *Serves* 1

1 tsp garlic-infused oil

Large pinch of asafoetida powder

1 tsp freshly grated ginger or ginger purée

8–9 large or approximately 100 g small prawns

1–2 stir-fry FODMAP-friendly vegetables of choice e.g. sliced bok choy/pak choi, sliced peppers, beansprouts, carrot batons, green part of spring onions, spinach leaves

1 packet of 'Straight to Wok' rice noodles or 1 dried nest or 150 g cooked rice noodles

1 tbsp oyster, soy, fish sauce to flavour

Heat the garlic-infused oil in a wok, and then stir in a pinch of asafoetida powder, and the fresh ginger or ginger purée. Add the prawns along with FODMAP-friendly vegetables and stir-fry for about 5–6 minutes. Add the cooked rice noodles and stir-fry for a further 3 minutes. Stir through the soy, fish or oyster sauce to flavour, adjust seasoning if needed and serve hot.

Coriander tuna steak and salad

Prep 5 mins. *Cook* 5 mins. *Serves* 1

Fresh tuna steak, 150 g

Salt and freshly ground black pepper

1 tbsp olive oil

Juice of 1 lime

Handful of fresh coriander leaves and stems, finely chopped

Green chilli, finely chopped and deseeded if desired

Season the tuna steak and drizzle with olive oil. Heat a non-stick frying pan over a medium heat. Rub the tuna with the lime juice, finely chopped coriander and chilli before cooking for 1 minute each side for rare, and 2 minutes for medium. Baste with the marinade as it cooks. Serve with FODMAP-friendly side salad of your choice and baked potato or basmati rice.

Mediterranean baked fish with wilted baby spinach

Prep 5 mins. *Cook* 20 mins. *Serves* 1

Fresh fillet of white fish, 150 g	***To serve:***
Salt and freshly ground pepper	*Jacket potato*
3–4 cherry tomatoes, halved	*Wilted baby spinach*
Handful of flat leaf parsley, chopped	*2 tsp FODMAP-friendly tartare sauce*

Preheat the oven to gas mark 5 / 190°C / 375°F. Season the fish and place in a tinfoil parcel large enough to hold the tomatoes. Lay the cherry tomatoes on top of the fish (count tomatoes as 1 fruit serving for the day). Sprinkle on the chopped flat leaf parsley and fold the foil to make a loose parcel. Place the parcel in an ovenproof dish and bake in for about 15–20 minutes until the fish is lightly cooked. Serve with baked potato, FODMAP-friendly wilted baby spinach and FODMAP-friendly tartare sauce.

Simply spiced salmon

Prep 5 mins. *Cook* 20 mins. *Serves* 1

Fresh fillet or steak of salmon

1 tsp chilli-infused oil

Spring onions (green stems only), finely sliced

Pinch of dried chilli flakes

Olive oil

To serve:

Boiled new potatoes or a baked potato, boiled rice or quinoa (microwave rice/quinoa pouches are convenient: ½ a pouch = 1 serving)

FODMAP-friendly vegetable of choice e.g. courgettes or carrots

Preheat the oven to gas mark 5 / 190°C / 375°F. Season the salmon with the chilli-infused oil, and sprinkle with finely sliced spring onion (green part only) and a pinch of chilli flakes. Drizzle with olive oil and wrap the spiced fish in tinfoil. Bake in the oven for about 20 minutes until lightly cooked. Serve with boiled new potatoes, a baked potato, boiled rice or quinoa and a FODMAP-friendly vegetable.

Chicken breast with fresh basil and Parmesan

Prep 15 mins. *Cook* 20 mins. *Serves* 1

1 chicken breast, about 150 g

Salt and coarsely ground black pepper

1–2 tsp basil-infused oil

4–6 new potatoes, as desired, or small tin of unpeeled Jersey Royals, drained

2 tsp olive oil

FODMAP-friendly vegetables of your choice e.g. baby spinach leaves and sliced courgettes

Parmesan cheese, as desired

Fresh basil leaves, torn

Preheat the oven to gas mark 5 / 190°C / 375°F. Season the chicken breast and drizzle with the basil-infused oil. Wrap this in foil and bake for about 20 minutes until the juices run clear. Meanwhile, if using fresh potatoes, boil the new potatoes until tender for about 15–20 minutes. Drain and set aside. If using canned potatoes, heat through in a little of the canning water. Heat the olive oil in a non-stick frying pan and sauté a mixture of FODMAP-friendly vegetables until just cooked. Add this to the cooked potatoes. Top with a sprinkle of grated Parmesan cheese and torn fresh basil leaves. Serve alongside the cooked, basil-infused chicken.

Chilli con carne

Prep 15 mins. *Cook* 20–30 mins. *Serves* 4

1½ tbsp of garlic- or chilli-infused oil

1 tsp asafoetida powder

500 g of lean minced beef, lamb, chicken or turkey

1 Maggi beef stock pot or Knorr Flavour Pot e.g. 3 Peppercorn (see Box, page 45)

Splash of Worcestershire sauce

2 tsp ground cumin

1 large carrot, finely chopped

2 sticks of celery, finely chopped

2 tbsp of tomato paste

1 tsp finely sliced fresh chilli or dried chilli flakes or lazy chilli purée of choice

400 g can of chopped tomatoes

Coarse black pepper

2 pouches microwave rice

25 g grated mozzarella cheese

Heat 1½ tbsp of garlic- or chilli-infused oil and if desired add 1 tsp asafoetida powder along with 500 g of lean minced beef, lamb, or turkey. Brown the mince on low heat for 3–4 minutes. Add the stock or Flavour Pot, a splash of Worcestershire sauce, 2 tsp ground cumin, 1 large finely chopped carrot and 2 sticks of finely chopped celery along with 2 tbsp of tomato paste and 1 tsp chilli of your choice. Stir for a few minutes on a medium heat. Add a large tin of chopped tomatoes. Season and simmer for about 20–30 minutes until the meat is tender. When the meat is nearly cooked, microwave the rice pouches. Sprinkle the cooked chill with a handful of grated mozzarella and serve with hot rice.

Variations

Serve with quinoa (microwave rice/quinoa pouches are convenient: ½ a pouch = 1 serving) OR in a corn taco shell OR with a baked potato alongside a FODMAP-friendly side salad of choice.

Chicken risotto with baby spinach and Parmesan

Prep 15 mins. *Cook* 25 mins. *Serves* 1

1 tsp garlic-infused oil

¼ tsp of asafoetida powder

Handful of spring onions (green part), finely sliced

1 chicken breast, cut into chunks

2 FODMAP-friendly vegetables of your choice e.g. ½ pepper sliced, finely sliced ¼ celery stalk, a handful of sliced green beans

75 g of Arborio risotto rice

300 ml chicken stock (see Box, page 45)

Handful of baby spinach

25 g Parmesan cheese

Freshly ground pepper

Heat 1 tsp garlic-infused oil along with a handful of finely sliced (green stems only) spring onion and ¼ tsp of asafoetida powder. Add the chunks of chicken breast and cook gently for 2–3 minutes. Add two FODMAP-friendly vegetables of your choice e.g. ½ pepper sliced, finely sliced ¼ celery stalk or a handful of sliced green beans. Stir-fry gently for 2–3 minutes. Stir in 75 g of the risotto rice and stir-fry gently for 2–3 minutes until the rice turns translucent. Add 300 ml of chicken stock to a measuring jug and pour a quarter of it into the pan. Stir continuously over a medium heat. Once all the liquid is absorbed, repeat this process until all the stock used up. Once all the stock is absorbed and the rice is cooked, add a generous handful of baby spinach and stir through. Sprinkle with a handful of Parmesan cheese, season with pepper and serve.

Spaghetti Bolognese

Prep 10 mins. Cook 35 mins. Serves 4

1½ tbsp of garlic-infused oil

1 tsp asafoetida powder

500 g of lean minced beef, lamb or turkey

1 Maggi beef stock pot or Knorr Mixed Herbs Flavour Pot (see Box, page 45)

Splash of Worcestershire sauce

1 large carrot, finely chopped

2 sticks of celery, finely chopped

2 tbsp of tomato paste

1–2 tsp of herbs of choice e.g. dried oregano, mixed herbs or basil

400 g can of chopped tomatoes

Coarse black pepper

25 g grated Parmesan cheese

300 g dried 'free from' spaghetti

Bacon rashers, finely sliced (optional)

Heat 1½ tbsp of garlic-infused oil and if you wish, add 1 tsp asafoetida powder along with 500 g of lean minced beef, lamb or turkey. Brown the mince over a low heat for 3–4 minutes. Add the stock or Flavour Pot, a splash of Worcestershire sauce, 1 large finely chopped carrot and 2 sticks of finely chopped celery. Stir-fry to blend the ingredients together. Add 2 tbsp of tomato paste and a teaspoon of herbs of your choice e.g. dried oregano, mixed herbs or basil. Stir for a few minutes on a medium heat. Add the tin of chopped tomatoes with the juices. Season, cover and simmer for about 30 minutes. Meanwhile, cook the 'free from' spaghetti until al dente. Serve the cooked Bolognese mince on top of a bed of spaghetti and sprinkle with a handful of grated Parmesan. For an enhanced meat flavour, you could also add a couple of finely sliced bacon rashers while the mince is browning.

Mexican corn tacos

Prep 10 mins. *Cook* 30 mins. *Serves* 4

1 tbsp garlic-infused oil

500 g of lean minced beef

Knorr 3 Peppercorn Flavour Pot (see Box, page 45)

Splash of Worcestershire sauce

Splash of chilli sauce

2 tsp ground coriander seeds

1 large carrot, finely chopped

2 sticks of celery, finely chopped

2 tbsp of tomato paste

1 tsp finely sliced fresh green chilli or dried chilli flakes or lazy chilli purée of choice

400 g can of chopped tomatoes

Coarse black pepper

8 corn taco shells

25 g grated mozzarella cheese

Handful flat leaf parsley, chopped

Heat the garlic-infused oil and add the 500 g of lean minced beef. Brown the mince on a low heat for 3–4 minutes. Add the 3 Peppercorn Flavour Pot, a splash of Worcestershire sauce, chilli sauce, ground coriander seeds, 1 large finely chopped carrot and 2 sticks of finely chopped celery along with 2 tbsp of tomato paste and 1 tsp chilli of your choice. Stir for a few minutes on a medium heat. Add the tin of chopped tomatoes. Season and simmer for about 20–30 minutes until the meat is tender. When the meat is cooked, spoon it into the taco shells. Sprinkle the cooked spicy mince with a handful of grated mozzarella and flat leaf parsley.

Vegetarian choices

Chilli con veggie

Prep 10 mins. *Cook* 20 mins. *Serves* 4

1½ tbsp of garlic- or chilli-infused oil

1 tsp asafoetida powder

500 g of Quorn mince

1 Knorr Mixed Herbs Flavour Pot
(see Box, page 45)

Splash of Worcestershire sauce

2 tsp ground cumin

1 large carrot, finely chopped

2 sticks of celery, finely chopped

2 tbsp of tomato paste

1 tsp finely sliced fresh chilli or
dried chilli flakes or lazy chilli
purée of choice

400 g can of lentils, drained
and rinsed

400 g can of chopped tomatoes

Coarse black pepper

2 pouches microwave rice

25 g grated mozzarella cheese

Heat 1½ tbsp of garlic- or chilli-infused oil and if desired add 1 tsp asafoetida powder along with 500 g of Quorn mince. Brown the mince over a low heat for 3–4 minutes. Add the Herbs Pot, a splash of Worcestershire sauce, ground cumin, 1 large finely chopped carrot and 2 sticks of finely chopped celery along with 2 tbsp of tomato paste and 1 tsp chilli of your choice. Stir for a few minutes on a medium heat. Add the tin of chopped tomatoes and the drained lentils. Season and simmer for about 15 minutes. When the Quorn is nearly cooked, microwave the rice pouches. Sprinkle the cooked veggie chill with a handful of grated mozzarella and serve with hot rice.

Spanish-style omelette

Prep 15 mins. *Cook* 15 mins. *Serves* 1

3–4 new potatoes, unpeeled

2 tsp olive oil

Handful of spring onions (green part only), finely sliced

40 g frozen petits pois

Handful of baby spinach leaves

2–3 eggs

25 g grated mature cheese

Salt and pepper, as desired

Freshly snipped chives (or 1 tsp dried)

Boil the new potatoes until tender, or for convenience use a small tin of Jersey Royals, drained. Heat the olive oil in a non-stick frying pan; add a generous handful of finely sliced spring onions (green part only), and fry gently until softened. Slice the cooked potatoes and add to the pan; fry for a couple of minutes, stirring gently so as not to break the potatoes too much. Stir in the frozen petit pois, or peas, along with handful of baby spinach leaves. Beat 2–3 eggs with the grated mature cheese. Season and pour over the potato mixture. Preheat the grill. Cook the egg in the pan over a low heat for about 5 minutes until the egg is just set. Place the pan under the preheated hot grill for 3–4 minutes to brown slightly and cook top. Scatter with dried or freshly cut chives and serve hot or cold.

Veggie Bolognese

Prep 10 mins. *Cook* 25–30 mins. *Serves* 4

1½ tbsp of garlic-infused oil

1 tsp asafoetida powder

500 g of Quorn mince

1 Knorr Mixed Herbs Flavour Pot (see Box, page 45)

Splash of Worcestershire sauce

1 large finely chopped carrot

2 sticks of finely chopped celery

2 tbsp of tomato paste

1–2 tsp of herbs of choice e.g. dried oregano, mixed herbs or basil

400 g can of chopped tomatoes

Coarse black pepper

25 g grated Parmesan cheese

300 g dried 'free from' spaghetti

To serve:

FODMAP-friendly side salad of your choice

Heat 1½ tbsp of garlic-infused oil and, if you wish, add 1 tsp asafoetida powder along with 500 g of Quorn mince. Brown the mince over a low heat for 3–4 minutes. Add the Flavour Pot, a splash of Worcestershire sauce, 1 large finely chopped carrot and 2 sticks of finely chopped celery. Stir-fry to blend the ingredients together. Add 2 tbsp of tomato paste and 1–2 tsp of herbs of your choice e.g. dried oregano, mixed herbs or basil. Stir for a few minutes on a medium heat. Add the tin of chopped tomatoes with the juices. Season, cover and simmer for about 15–20 minutes. Meanwhile, cook the 'free from' spaghetti until *al dente*. Serve the cooked Quorn mince on top of a bed of spaghetti alongside the side salad, and sprinkle with a handful of grated Parmesan. Alternatively, eat with quinoa or a baked potato. To bulk out the Bolognese, you could also add 1 x 400 g can of drained and rinsed lentils.

Time to bake

FODMAP-friendly scones

Prep 15 mins. *Cook* 20 mins. *Makes* 6–8

230 g gluten-free self-raising flour

2 tsp of xanthum gum

1 level tsp of baking powder

60 g of soft margarine

1 dessertspoonful of ground chia seeds (optional)

1 egg, beaten and made up to 150 ml with lactose-free milk

Preheat the oven to gas mark 6 / 200°C / 400°F. Add the flour, xanthum gum, baking powder and margarine to a large mixing bowl. Add a dessertspoonful of ground chia seeds if desired. Break the egg into a measuring jug and top up to 150 ml with lactose-free milk. Beat the two together and add to the dry ingredients in the mixing bowl. Finally, gently mix all the ingredients with a hand blender or food processor. Drop the dough onto a floured surface and shape into 6–8 balls. Flatten out with your hand or a rolling pin until about 2 cm thick and then, using a cutter, cut out your scones. Brush the tops with a spot of lactose-free milk. Pop the scones onto a greased baking tray and place in the preheated oven for 15–20 minutes.

Suitable for freezing.

Oat cookies

Prep 15 mins. *Cook* 15 mins. *Makes* 8–10

115 g soft margarine	***Optional extras:***
85 g caster sugar	*Add 1 tbsp of chia seeds*
1 tbsp golden syrup	*Add 1 dessertspoon of cocoa*
115 g of rolled oats	*powder*
115 g gluten-free self-raising flour	
1 egg	

Preheat the oven to gas mark 4 / 180°C / 350°F. Add all the ingredients to a large mixing bowl and mix together with a beater or food processor. (Add any of the optional extras before beating.) Take a small handful of the mixture and roll into a golf ball-size round and shape into a cookie. Place this onto a greased baking sheet and flatten the cookie gently with a fork. Repeat for the rest of the dough. Bake in the centre of the oven for 15 minutes. Cool on a wire rack and store in an airtight container for up to 24 hrs.

Chocolate chip cookies

Prep 15 mins. *Cook* 15 mins. *Makes* 8–10

115 g soft margarine

85 g caster sugar

1 tbsp golden syrup

115 g of rolled oats

115 g gluten-free self-raising flour

1 dessertspoon of cocoa powder

100 g bag of chocolate chips

1 egg, beaten

Preheat the oven to gas mark 4 / 180°C / 350°F. Mix all the dry ingredients together in a large mixing bowl, then add the beaten egg and blend using a beater or food processor. Take a small handful of the mixture and roll into a golf ball-size round and shape into a cookie. Place this onto a greased baking sheet and flatten the cookie gently with a fork. Repeat for the rest of the dough. Bake in the centre of the oven for 15 minutes. Cool on a wire rack and store in an airtight container for up to 24 hrs.

Low-FODMAP pancakes

Prep 10 mins. *Cook* 15 mins. *Makes* 6–7 pancakes

100 g of gluten-free self-raising flour

25 g of sugar (omit if making savoury pancakes)

1 egg, beaten and made up to 300 ml with lactose-free milk

1–2 tsp chia seeds (optional)

Spray oil or 1–2 tbsp vegetable oil e.g. rapeseed for frying

To serve:

Drizzle of lemon juice or sliced strawberries or blueberries

Sift the flour in to a large bowl. Stir in the sugar, if making sweet pancakes. Gradually add the egg and milk mixture to the flour and sugar with a hand blender or whisk until the batter is smooth. If you wish at this stage you can sprinkle in 1–2 tsp of chia seeds for a protein and fibre boost! Heat a drizzle of vegetable oil in a non-stick frying pan. Once the oil is hot, wipe the pan with a piece of kitchen paper to mop up the excess and pour in the first ladle of batter. Cook gently and flip over once the mixture starts to bubble. Cook for a further 1–2 minutes on the other side before serving. Add a little more oil to the pan and wipe the excess, as before,with a piece of kitchen paper. Continue to add 1 ladle of the batter at a time until the mixture is used up. You should be able to make 6–7 pancakes. Serve immediately or store in an airtight container for up to 24 hrs or they can be frozen for another day. Serve with a favourite low-FODMAP topping, sweet or savoury, e.g. a drizzle of lemon juice or sliced strawberries/blueberries.

Hungry between meals?

Snacking can be helpful, or unhelpful, depending on the foods we choose. A planned, strategic snack can help us keep to regular, wise eating habits, especially if we have long periods, e.g. more than 4–5 hours, between meals. There's nothing like feeling ravenous to trigger mindless grabbing at whatever we can get our hands on to keep going. Everyone will have different snacking preferences, but a helpful guide is to have 3 regular meals and 1–2 planned snacks each day, ensuring the snacks are part of our day's overall eating plan. Planning helps us to have the right foods to hand, and stay away from convenience snack foods. It also helps us stay on track with our eating habits by knowing that a snack is coming before too long. If you need to snack on the go and won't have access to good choices, then choose easily transportable snacks and pack them in your bag (put them into a small container if need be) before you leave the house.

Fifteen flavoursome snack ideas

1 FODMAP-friendly 'gluten-free/free from' pancakes or home-made pancakes topped with a savoury or sweet choice (see recipe, page 66)
2 FODMAP-friendly 'gluten-free/free from' crackers or oatcakes and cheese
3 Free from scone (see recipe, page 62) and a spread of FODMAP-friendly jam
4 Rice cakes and peanut butter topped with sliced banana
5 Handful of FODMAP-friendly unsalted nuts and/or seeds
6 Peanut 9Bar (check label)
7 FODMAP-friendly vegetable sticks and lactose-free cream cheese
8 Carrot or cucumber batons with a few olives (avoid olives flavoured with garlic)
9 Glass of lactose-free milk and banana
10 FODMAP-friendly 'gluten-free/free from' toast with peanut butter and sliced banana
11 Dark chocolate chunks
12 FODMAP-friendly fruit (see ideas in the breakfast ideas section, page 42; 1 serving only up to max of 3 per day)

13 Handful of small olives; approximately 15 (avoid olives in garlic)

14 Potato crisps: plain or salt and vinegar are generally suitable

15 Homemade or FODMAP-friendly shop-bought popcorn (plain, sweet or salted popcorn).

Note that not all gluten-free/free from products will be FODMAP friendly. Savoury and sweet snacks often contain some FODMAP ingredients, commonly: honey, agave nectar, fructose, inulin, fruit juice concentrate, apple juice, wheat, rye, barley, onion and garlic.

Homemade popcorn

Prep 5 mins. *Cook* 5 mins. *Serves* 4–6

1 tbsp cooking oil e.g. rapeseed oil	*Flavouring:*
Small handful of popping corn kernels	*e.g. sprinkling of salt, sugar, sweetener, dried red chilli powder*

Gently heat 1 tbsp of cooking oil in a large pan and add a small handful of popping corn kernels. Cover the pan with a lid and heat the kernels gently; they will start popping in a few minutes. Keep the lid on tightly until you can count about 2 seconds in-between each pop. Remove the pan from the heat and transfer your popcorn into a bowl. One serving is about 20 g or a small bowl. Sprinkle with salt, sugar, sweetener or dried red chilli powder.

Index

adrenalin, for anaphylaxis 13
alcohol 20
allergies *see* food allergies
alverine 26
anaphylaxis, food allergies and 12–13

bacteria, normal bowel 2
biscodyl 27
bladder, irritable 8
bleeding
  causes of 8
  IBS as cause of 29–30
  as warning sign 4
blood tests
  diagnosis of IBS 15, 16
bowel, large
  anatomy and function of 1–3
  gas 5
  gastrocolic reflex 5
  gurgling 5
  warning/red flag signs 4
bowel movements
  changes in 8
  stool samples 17
  types of 3–5
butternut squash or sweet potato soup 46

caffeine 20
campylobacter 32
cancer
  IBS and 29–30
  ovarian 8–9
  rectal 8–9
carrot and coriander soup 45
celeriac allergy 13
celery allergy 13
chicken breast with fresh basil and Parmesan 54
chicken risotto with baby spinach and Parmesan 56
chilli con carne 55
chilli con veggie 59

chocolate chip cookies 64
cognitive behavioural therapy 26
colonoscopy 17–18
constipation
  food intolerance 11
  range of movements 3–5
  as warning sign 4
coriander tuna steak and salad 51
counselling
  for stress 25–6

diarrhoea
  food intolerances 11
  as warning sign 4
diet and nutrition *see also* low-FODMAP diet
  managing IBS 19–22
  recipes 42–67

egg allergy 13
exercise
  finding interest in 23–4
  managing IBS and 19, 23–5
  maximum heart rate 24–5

fatigue 8
fibre 21–2
fish and seafood recipes
  coriander tuna steak and salad 51
  fish noodle supper 49
  Mediterranean baked fish 52
  simply spiced salmon 53
  Singapore-style prawn noodles 50
fish noodle supper 49
fizzy drinks 21
flatulence and bloating
  food intolerances 11
  as symptom of IBS 7–9
  trouble foods 21
FODMAP *see* low-FODMAP diet
food allergies
  anaphylaxis and 12–13

causes of 12
cooking eggs 13
oral 13
symptoms of 12–13
testing for 14
types of 12
food diary
for diagnosis of IBS 15
managing IBS 19
food intolerances 11–12
fried/fatty food 20, 21
fructan 29
fructose 22, 31, 34

gas *see* flatulence and bloating
gastrocolic reflex 5
gluten-free eating 36, 40–1
baking recipes 62–5
low-FODMAP pancakes 65
snacks 66–7

headache 8
heartburn 8
hormones
IBS and 15, 19
hyoscine 26

immune system
allergies and 12
intolerances, food 11–12
irritable bowel syndrome (IBS)
bowel function and 1–3
diagnosis of 15–18
exercise and 23–5
incidence of 7
length of symptoms 29
long-term effects of 29
managing diet and 19–22
medical recognition of ix–x
medications for 26–7
post-infectious 30
stress and 25–6
symptoms of 7–9
ispaghula husk 27
itching
food allergies and 12

King's College, London
develops FODMAP diet 31–2

lactose
FODMAP foods 34
IBS and intolerance 29
lactulose 27
low-FODMAP diet
baking and treats 62–7
breakfast 41–3
condiments and flavourings 39–40
definition and development 31–2
diary and cheeses 37
fats and sugars 38–9
foods to avoid 34
fruit and vegetables 35, 38, 41–2
grains and starches 36
lunches 43–8
main meals 49–61
protein sources 36–7
shopping list 34–40
snacks 39
stock cubes 35, 39, 45
tips for baking 40–1

macrogols 27
mannitol 34
maximum heart rate 24–5
meat and poultry recipes
chicken breast with fresh basil and
Parmesan 54
chicken risotto with baby spinach
and Parmesan 56
chilli con carne 55
Mexican corn tacos 58
spaghetti Bolognese 57
mebeverine 26
medication
anti-depressants 26, 27
anti-diarrhoeals 26, 27
anti-spasmodics 26
laxatives 26–7
managing IBS 19
Mediterranean baked fish with wilted
baby spinach 52
menstrual cycles
food diary and 19
IBS and 15
methylcellulose 27
Mexican corn tacos 58
milk
allergy to 13

lactose intolerance 11
Monash University
    FODMAP diet app 33, 35, 40
muscle pain 8

nausea 8
nut allergy 13

oat cookies 63
oats 41
onion and garlic 34–5
ovarian cancer 8–9

pain
    food intolerances 11
    as symptom of IBS 7–9
    as warning sign 4
pancake recipe 65
peppermint oil 26
physical examination for IBS 16
popcorn recipe 68
probiotics 22
processed foods 20, 21

raffinose 32
rashes, food allergies and 12
roasted red pepper soup 48

salmonella 30
scone recipe 62
selective serotonin re-uptake
    inhibitors (SSRIs) 27
senna 27
shellfish allergy 13

shigella 32
sigmoidoscopy 17
simply spiced salmon 53
Singapore-style prawn noodles
    50
sorbitol 32, 34
soup recipes
    butternut squash or sweet potato
    46
    carrot and coriander 45
    roasted red pepper 48
    tomato and basil 47
spaghetti Bolognese 57
Spanish-style omelette 60
squash soup 46
stool samples 17
stress 19, 25–6
sweet potato soup 46

tomato and basil soup 47
tricyclic anti-depressants 27

vegetarian recipes
    chilli con veggie 59
    Spanish-style omelette 60
    veggie Bolognese 61
veggie Bolognese 61
vitamins, gut bacteria and 2

weight loss 4

X-rays 18
xanthan gum 41
xylitol 34